INSANITY DEFENSE

INSANITY DEFENSE

by

RICHARD ARENS

With a Foreword by

HAROLD D. LASSWELL

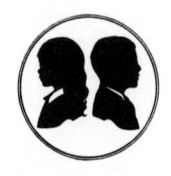

PHILOSOPHICAL LIBRARY
New York

Copyright, © 1974, by Philosophical Library, Inc.,
15 East 40th Street, New York, N. Y. 10016

All rights reserved

Library of Congress Catalog Card No. 72-96108
SBN 8022-2106-8

Manufactured in the United States of America

TO THE MEMORY OF

MYRON G. EHRLICH

We must be very cautious; it is not every frantic and idle humour of a man, that would exempt him from justice, and the punishment of the law. . . . A mad man as is to be exempted from punishment . . . must be a man that is totally deprived of his understanding and memory and doth not know what he is doing, no more than an infant, than a brute, or a wild beast. . . .

The Wild Beast Test

It must be clearly proved that . . . the party accused was labouring under such a defect of reason, from disease of the mind, as not to know the nature and quality of the act he was doing; or if he did know it that he did not know he was doing what was wrong.

The M'Naghten Rules

And be these juggling fiends no more believ'd,
That palter with us in a double sense,
That keep the word of promise to our ear,
And break it to our hope.

Macbeth

FOREWORD

Professor Arens has written an illuminating study of an innovation that failed. The innovation was a judicial doctrine of criminal responsibility;[1] the failure was to effect a stable change in the behavior of the institutions concerned.

In what sense was the *Durham* rule an innovation? It was undoubtedly a novelty in the District of Columbia in 1954 when it was enunciated. However, the fundamental principle was well-known elsewhere.[2] Seen in the larger context, Professor Arens is analyzing an instance of doctrinal diffusion rather than of independent innovation. Nonetheless it is pertinent to note that the enunciation of the formula gave great visibility to a policy that had made little headway in other jurisdictions.

It is not within the scope of Professor Arens' report to account for the response of the court, and to explain why the decision came in the early fifties. Without going into detail it can at least be said that the *Durham* rule reflected an expanding psychiatric ideology in the United States. Psychiatric theories had received a great boost when Sigmund Freud's psychoanalysis attracted the attention of literary men, and achieved both popularity and notoriety in mass media of dissemination. Academic psychology and

---

[1] Durham v. United States, 214 F.2d 862 (D.C. Cir. 1954) postulated non-responsibility whenever the "unlawful act was the product of mental disease or mental defect."
[2] *See* State v. Jones, 50 N.H. 369, 372-373 (1871); State v. Pike, 49 N.H. 399 (1869). For a survey of some of the intellectual history underlying the New Hampshire rule, see L. E. REIK *The Doe-Ray Correspondence: A Pioneer Collaboration In the Jurisprudence of Mental Disease,* 63 YALE L. J. 183 (1953).

psychiatry were ultimately affected and, reinforced by public curiosity, made up for lost time.[3] World War II precipitated a tremendous growth of psychiatrically trained personnel, and contributed to the acceptance of conceptions of mental illness that went beyond the organic characteristics of the individual to include difficulties that arise from unresolved value conflicts. A side effect of the preoccupation with mental illness was impatience with the courts, especially with the *monstrous practice of punishing a product of illness*. The proper function of ordinary sanctioning, it is widely sensed or said, is to deal with deviations that result from the calculated risks undertaken by healthy people.

The District of Columbia Court accepted the "product rule" in place of the traditional "knowledge rule." The obvious question is what the difference would have been if the *Durham* innovation had succeeded. First, defendants whose deviational acts were "the product of mental illness," whether classified as "psychotic" or "neurotic," would not have been held criminally responsible. Second, arrangements would have been made by the courts for nonresponsible offenders to obtain medical treatment under circumstances in which they would endanger neither themselves nor others. If hospital care was indicated, the hospitals would have had at their disposal the facilities necessary to use the therapeutic measures required to overcome the illness. If hospital confinement was not necessary, therapy would be provided outside the institution. If the patient did not yield to therapy, and indefinite custody was imperative the court would regularly supervise the conditions under which the patient lived, with a view to ensuring his greatest feasible degree of participation in society.[4]

[3] D. SHAKOW and D. RAPAPORT, THE INFLUENCE OF FREUD ON AMERICAN PSYCHOLOGY (1964).
[4] From this perspective, success of the *Durham* innovation would have required a doctrinal development—far beyond the scope of extant Durham jurisprudence—to say nothing of the requisite development of human and material resources. *See generally* DESSION, *Psychiatry and the Conditioning of Criminal Justice,* 47 YALE L.J. 319 (1938).

Professor Arens shows how far the actual course of events diverged from this set of potential results. It is quite clear that to some extent judges, jurors and attorneys were averse to enlarging the scope of the "insanity defense," especially if the defendants failed to conform to popular images of "craziness"; and were simply "neurotic." To some extent government psychiatrists in the District of Columbia were abashed by the magnitude of the burden that might have been placed on them, and cooperated in restricting the scope of the plea. Public psychiatric hospitals were acutely short of the means required to provide adequate therapy. Although they did not take an initiative to widen the insanity defense, they nevertheless found it expedient to act as though they were equipped to meet current demands to treat committed offenders. Hence they acquiesced in policies that progressively transformed hospitals into prisons. As the true state of affairs became more widely known, lawyers and others who initially welcomed the innovation saw that under the circumstances it was becoming a means of denying human rights.

The *Durham* episode calls attention to the inadequate institutions now available in Washington, D.C., and in many other jurisdictions in the United States, for the administration of justice. Strictly speaking, American public order is not organized to do the job at any level. The prosecuting attorney is indeed a "prosecutor," and admonitions to do evenhanded justice cannot often change his spots. Fortunately, we are making some headway toward introducing public defenders. However, these officials are usually overburdened with pressing cases. The role of a police commissioner is stereotyped by conventional expectations; so, too, is that of a commissioner of corrections. And a health commissioner, or superintendent of hospitals, cannot be expected to have a balanced and realistic view of those who are turned over to him as an alternative to prison.

The long and short of it is that it is nobody's official duty to provide a comprehensive picture of the administration of justice in any American jurisdiction. Hence there is no one to speak out and claim that if one million dollars is added to the hospital budget, the five per cent (?) who now obtain satisfactory therapy can be increased to fifty per cent; or that for two million dollars the percentage could increase to eighty. There is no one to propose that if the hospitals are inadequate, the "nonresponsible criminals" should be released or kept in a new type of correctional institution where their predicament can be kept more visible than when they are merged in hospital-prisons or the prison-hospitals.[5]

Perhaps a secretary of state for justice, or his counterpart at lower levels, is needed in American Government. Or, if this innovation is too disturbing to conventional perspectives, the emerging office of ombudsman might be charged with responsibility for preparing a report annually on the functioning of the judicial process as a whole, coupled with recommendations. In this way the function of review (appraisal) could be strengthened, and a centripetal force introduced into the fragmented American system.

Professor Arens' report is, in fact, a privately sponsored appraisal of official agencies in reference to one policy innovation. The initiative for the study was taken by civic-minded citizens who hoped that the *Durham* rule would mark a permanent advance in sanction law. The funds came from a private foundation and from public sources; and the project was administered by a board appointed by a private institution devoted to psychiatric teaching, research and consultation.

---

[5] The proposal that "nonresponsible criminals" have a "right to treatment" and that they should be released if the hospital in which they are placed is inadequate has, in fact, been entertained and has acquired the status of legal doctrine in the District of Columbia. *See* Rouse v. Cameron, 373 F.2d 451 (D.C. Cir. 1966). As a practical matter, however, at the time that this is written, the enforcement of the right to treatment in the District Court appears illusory and the Court of Appeals does not appear anxious to translate stated aspirations into operational realities. *See* Rouse v. Cameron, 387 F.2d 241 (D.C. Cir. 1967).

In some ways the most interesting feature of the research was the opportunity that it gave for actual participation in the everyday administration of criminal justice. Arens was a member of the bar, and the original plan was to select clients who were in need of aid, and whose situation raised important problems in law and psychiatry. It might be assumed by the outsider that public officials would welcome a civic-minded participant-observer. Such an assumption would greatly underestimate the intensity of the views that prevailed in many professional as well as lay quarters about the "coddling" of criminals and the unwelcome competition that was perceived as coming from psychiatrists in the disposition of offenders. Some officials began to be uncooperative and difficulties slowly multiplied. The members of the project board were prominent and busy people; hence it is little wonder that at first they did not realistically assess the resistances in the situation; hence resistances began to harden. Although the original program was not completed as planned, the results obtained are sufficiently representative to provide a valuable picture of the balance of factors—personal, professional, organizational—that ultimately blocked the innovation.

The vehemence of the conflict precipitated by the *Durham* doctrine, complicated as it was by other than intellectual considerations, gained much of its resonance from the unsettled, problematic character of the issues involved. There is, of course, broad verbal consensus on the proposition that people ought not to be punished for the "crime" of being sick. Such a standard is comparatively simple to apply when an organic defect is involved of a type that medical experts are agreed in diagnosing. The testimony of experts on organic conditions is usually treated with deference; or at least with greater respect than testimony about "functional" mental diseases. Lay jurors, judges and counsellors at law are reluctant to believe that a person who is entirely aware that he is doing wrong is nevertheless driven to perform a forbidden act as a result of conflicting drives of whose nature he is unaware. The situation is further confounded when a finding of nonresponsibility by reason of mental illness may result in curtailing the freedom of the defendant indefinitely—until physicians persuade the court that therapy has succeeded, or that the chances are low that the individual will ever again find himself in such provocative circumstances that he will be a menace to himself or others.

The ambiguities in the situation are exaggerated by the indirect fashion in which pertinent issues are conventionally framed. First of all, a moment's reflection confirms the point that a decision is always future oriented; that is, the consequences of the disposition of an offender are always in the future. This is true of the "deterrence" effect on the conduct of others. It applies to the "restoration" of whatever can be reinstated of the damage done by the offender. It is applicable to "rehabilitation," and to the "prevention" of provocative situations. Despite the future incidence of these consequences, the discussion of the future is usually cursory, overcondensed or indirect. Among the pertinent questions might be the following: (a) If released, is it likely that the offender's mental illness will operate significantly to produce offenses of a similar, an aggravated, or an attenuated character? (b) If therapy is indicated, can this be carried on without removing the patient from ordinary life? (c) If the illness cannot be cured, what is the minimum degree of removal from ordinary life that will protect the individual and the community from a serious degree of danger? Clearly, public policy requires that community decision makers be authorized to make these determinations, and that they have the benefit of the best guesses available. Since the limits of "sickness" are poorly defined, it is entirely appropriate that community decision makers examine the expert sufficiently to provide some understanding of the phenomena on which his inferences are based. A decision maker does not act rationally if he tries to substitute his judgment for the expert's; but he does proceed sensibly if he goes far enough to comprehend why experts disagree, and to see what the technical disagreements add up to in terms of the future behavior of the offender.

Our standard decision process provides for a complex interplay between nonexpert laymen and experts who advise laymen and one another. The juror, for instance, is usually a layman, but he too may happen to have specialized knowledge pertinent to the cases before him. The parties are represented by legal experts and may use psychiatric and other knowledgeable witnesses; and a judge may utilize specialists of his own. Obviously, our judicial system gives deference to the familiar maxim that experts should be on "tap," not on "top." It also allows for more education of jurors (and of new judges and lawyers) than is usually provided for. Why not arrange for pretrial education of prospective jurors (as well as for new members of the bar)?

At first sight it might seem wasteful to re-educate every panel of jurors in criminal cases to the prevailing wisdom about mental disease. This depends on the depth of shared concern for informed justice. Modern means of communication put in our hands the means of transmitting a great deal of information quickly and vividly to adults as well as children. The judges in a jurisdiction might, for instance, take responsibility for educational films that would introduce prospective jurors to contemporary conceptions of mental illness. The films could be selected or prepared under the auspices of bar and medical associations, or of professional schools. Many existing films are eligible for inclusion in such a training program.

It is of interest to social scientists and students of legal process generally that Professor Arens used a specific research approach. It is most accurate to think of it as a form of "prototyping," rather than of "experimentation" or "intervention."[6] The principal purpose was to enlighten us

―――――――

[6] *See* R.R. RUBENSTEIN AND H.D. LASSWELL, THE SHARING OF POWER IN A PSYCHIATRIC HOSPITAL, ch. 11 (1966).

about the conditions affecting the success of doctrinal innovation in law, with particular reference to sanction law. The project was not a true experiment; it arranged no controls, and formulated no theoretical model in advance. Nor was the project an intervention, since it was not from the beginning a matter of big time politics, like the anti-poverty program. We speak of an intervention when power considerations are so prominent that control passes out of the hands of those who are primarily concerned with the advancement of knowledge. When the Arens program began to arouse large scale controversy, it was probably wise to terminate it from a pure research perspective, since the principal features of the Washington situation had become abundantly clear. The strategy of selective participation in an ordinary institutional setting—which is prototyping—had already paid off. The research project served as a probe that revealed the direction and intensity of relevant predispositions.

Seen in conjunction with other studies the results reported in this book can be used to develop flexible yet realistic strategies for introducing effective changes into the administration of justice, which is the field of sanction law. The dissemination of the present report is a step in the process of appraisal that in turn leads to planning. The *Durham* experience may be widely understood to cast doubt on the efficacy of doctrinal innovations which, if taken literally, arouse non-cooperation among an overwhelming number of those who are most immediately concerned in the everyday administration of justice. Instead of new doctrine more may perhaps be accomplished by the modernization of old doctrines, especially when conjoined with pretrial education in contemporary conceptions of mental health and disease. For instance, the old "knowledge rule" can be properly reinterpreted to distinguish between types and degrees of knowledge. The range is from *designative* perceptions to those we can identify as *prescriptive*. The former are descriptive; the latter are normative and imperative. The mental condition of the individual does not permit him to accept the latter perceptions as vividly credible guides to *immediate* conduct. Merely *descriptive* (designative) perceptions are possible; prescriptive perceptions are precluded. And *prescriptive knowledge,* not simple designative knowledge, is what is pertinent to conduct, and to law. It is prescriptive knowledge of norms that is interfered with by mental disease. The old knowledge rule, in competent hands, is a prescriptive knowledge rule.

Among other possible changes would be the requirement of a pretrial showing by public authorities of responsibility for an offensive act.[7] In our creative age this does not exhaust the list.

I strongly suspect that this report will stimulate the psychiatric profession to accelerate the reconsideration of its own role in law and society.

This would indeed be a landmark if it stimulates lawyers and physicians, as well as attentive citizens, to perceive that our American Government is not organized to live up to our verbal commitment to human dignity in the administration of justice, especially to a sick offender.

HAROLD D. LASSWELL
Ford Foundation Professor Emeritus
of Law and the Social Sciences, Yale University;
Distinguished Visiting Professor of Law and History,
Temple University

---

[7] *See* Goldstein and Katz, *Abolish the Insanity Defense, Why Not?* 72 YALE L. J. 853 (1963).

CONTENTS

	Foreword	ix
	Acknowledgments	xxi
	Prologue	xxiii
Chapter I	Durham and its Challenge	1
II	A Short History of a Project in Insanity Research and Litigation	19
III	Judicial Psychiatry and Psychiatric Justice	29
IV	Due Process and the Rights of the Mentally Ill: The Strange Case of Frederick Lynch	83
V	The Quest for the Impartial Psychiatric Expert: Reality and Illusion in the Insanity Defense	103
VI	The Defense of Walter X. Wilson: An Insanity Plea and a Skirmish in the War on Poverty	143
VII	Heresy in the Courtroom: The Defense of a Drug Addict as Mentally Ill	221
	Epilogue — Back to Methuselah	289
	Appendix I	305
	Appendix II	311
	Appendix III	327

ACKNOWLEDGMENTS

Professor Harold D. Lasswell read the entire manuscript in its various stages of development and provided a powerful combination of encouragement and constructive criticism, essential to whatever emerged as valuable in this book.

Father David Granfield of the Catholic University Law Faculty remained an unfailing friend, critic and supporter on the arduous road from first draft to publication with the Philosophical Library and beyond it.

Mr. Colman Stein of the District of Columbia bar rendered lonely but effective moral and political support to an often unpopular cause in the inner councils of the Washington School of Psychiatry for which I can never express full gratitude.

More lawyers than there is space to acknowledge rallied to the support of a project, attacked for furnishing free legal and psychiatric aid to the mentally disordered indigent defendants in the criminal courts. Equal numbers among them rallied to the support of their own clients under like handicaps and with like assistance—often at considerable professional cost—none with greater personal courage and dedication than the late Myron G. Ehrlich.

Dr. Charles E. Goshen, formerly of the District of Columbia, and now Professor of Psychiatry at Vanderbilt University, gave generously of his time and advice throughout years of tempestuous and at times hazardous litigation and research.

Both McGill University and the University of Toronto furnished a supportive atmosphere in the best tradition of academic freedom for the completion and revision of the work.

I am further indebted to Mr. Patrick Horgan, a graduate student at the Osgoode Hall Law School, York University and Mr. T.S. Robbins, an undergraduate student at the University of Toronto Law Faculty, both of whom rendered valuable and indeed essential editorial assistance.

All are of course to be absolved from the limitation of the work.

Law and Society, The Catholic University Law Review, The Villanova Law Review and *The Howard Law Journal* graciously permitted publication of some of my work.

R. A.

PROLOGUE

In the first glow generated by the Warren Court and less than a year before the issuance of the order for the desegregation of the nation's public schools in *Brown v. Board of Education*[1] the Court of Appeals for the District of Columbia Circuit proclaimed the discovery of a rule of reason for the differentiation between "bad men" and "sick men." It declared in *Durham v. United States* that punishment could not be imposed for behavior which was the product of mental disorder.[2]

Dr. Karl Menninger hailed this development as more significant than the desegregation decision of the Supreme Court and his acclaim of the new insanity rule in the District of Columbia was joined in by most official spokesmen of American psychiatry.

Numerous attempts had in fact been made in the courts —before *Durham*—to afford the stringent "right-wrong test" of *M'Naghten* a degree of flexibility not altogether inconsistent with expanding intellectual horizons. Most had been frustrated by a congeries of obstacles exemplified by the nemesistic—if not clinically sadistic—inclination of wide strata of decision-makers, the pressures of a prosecution bent upon its pound of flesh and a general lack of syntactical sophistication of the trial bench. A bad situation was compounded by the inability of the impoverished defendant to secure the appropriately skilled alienist, capable of transmit-

---

[1] 349 U.S. 294 (1955).
[2] Durham v. United States, 214 F. 2d 862 (D.C. Cir. 1954).

ting a concern for the life of his patient, in meaningful terms to a lay jury.

Durham was seen as the dawn of a new day. Psychiatrists were directed to proceed within wider horizons of knowledge and invited to prevent the monstrous practice of punishing the product of mental disorder. They were called upon to raise the level of legal-psychiatric collaboration to the point where it would be accessible to rich and poor alike. They failed miserably—"fouling up the legal process"—as expressed by Dr. Karl Menninger. And so did the judges, explicitly "for want of trying," despite the disclaimer of Bazelon, C.J.

A project exploring the operations of the new rule starting in 1959 and continuing, "not without interruption," beyond the mid-sixties found that after an initial attempt at *bona fide* experimentation, judicial and psychiatric decisionmakers returned to ancient and more familiar ways. *M'Naghten* had received judicial burial—but it continued to rule the criminal courts from its grave. So, indeed, did an even more ancient judicial criterion of criminal responsibility: the wild beast test.

In a word, the District of Columbia judiciary—sustained and supported by the men in white—maintained the monstrous practice of punishing the product of mental illness while continuing to pay lip service to a rule reflective of the reason and compassion of 1954.

The report of the project as embodied in this book, describes the scene through the middle sixties.

Nothing, however, has changed for the better since that time. Lingering hopes for a resurgence of judicial conscience were dashed when the Durham Court sought the explicit exorcism of even the ghost of its own rule by adopting the *Brawner* doctrine—not significantly distinguishable from *M'Naghten* in its most rigid 19th century sense.

The impoverished defendant suffering from mental illness is thus stripped of every scrap of hope. He had long despaired of government psychiatry. He has now been shaken in a vital article of American faith, the belief that at least "the courts would stand against any winds that blow as havens of refuge for those who might otherwise suffer because they are helpless, weak, outnumbered or because they are nonconforming victims of prejudice and public excitement."[3]

The system—as seen by some of its victims—appears dismal and essentially radicalizing:

> "That pack of scoundrels
> Tumbling through the gate
> Emerges
> As the Order
> Of the State."[4]

---

[3] Mr. Justice Black, for the Court, in Chambers v. Florida, 309 U.S. 227, 241 (1940).
[4] S. KUNITZ, THE TESTING TREE (1971).

Chapter I

DURHAM AND ITS CHALLENGE

THE PRIMARY QUESTION

Irrespective of recent reforms, our penal law has continued to reflect a dominant spirit of crudely retributive justice.[1] Whatever the improvements of the contemporary system of criminal justice, they have not been of an order to bring about a substantial reorientation of basic purposes or to remove the sting from Edmund Burke's observation—if it be applied to our system of justice:

> In the groves of *their* academy, at the end of every vista you see nothing but the gallows.[2]

Any attempt at the replacement of traditional criminal sanctions by sanction-equivalents, rationally and humanely designed to achieve the rehabilitation of the "criminal," can be hailed as a significant upward step in man's long and arduous quest for a civilized code of correction.[3] Such a step was seen by men of good will in an action of the United

---

[1] For a documentation of this theme *see* R. ARENS AND H.D. LASSWELL, IN DEFENSE OF PUBLIC ORDER, 24-107, 128-130 (1961).

[2] E. BURKE, III THE WORKS OF EDMUND BURKE 33 (London, John C. Nimmo Publishers, 1887).

[3] The term *sanction-equivalents* was coined by the late Professor George H. Dession. He defined sanction-equivalents as "nondepriving ways of coping with the actual or threatened flouting of a prescription . . ." Dession, *Deviation and Community Sanctions in* PSYCHIATRY AND LAW (Hoch and Zubin, ed. 1955). Such sanction-equivalents might include but would by no means be restricted to psychotherapy, a welfare program and the whole host of instrumentalities recently devised in the "war on poverty."

States Court of Appeals for the District of Columbia in 1954. *Durham v. United States*[4] provided for the imposition of what appeared at first glance to be a civilized system of psychiatric sanction-equivalents in *lieu* of conventional punishment in any case in which the crime appeared to be a product of mental disorder. The rule seemed premised upon the assumption that it was both wrong and foolish to punish where punishment could not correct and where remedial measures of a medical or quasi-medical kind could assure both the affected individual and society of any reasonable probability of nonrecurrence of the "criminal" event which triggered social intervention.[5] In a word, the new rule rejected the punishment of any act which was the product of mental disorder.[6]

Practising lawyers in the District of Columbia saw the rule almost intuitively as inviting compassion as well as a more careful and comprehensive scientific assessment of an element of crime, hitherto conspicuously and irrationally neglected in too many cases—the mental state of the accused.[7] The court itself seemed to strive to make facilities for the exploration of the insanity defense available to all who sought them—though essentially only at the hands of government psychiatrists.[8]

[4] Durham v. United States, 214 F.2d 862 (D.C. Cir. 1954).

[5] Thus the Court of Appeals for the District of Columbia declared: "It is both wrong and foolish to punish where there is no blame and where punishment cannot correct." Williams v. United States, 250 F.2d 19 (D.C. Cir. 1957). For some of my views of rational sanction alternatives developed with Professor Harold D. Lasswell, *see* Lasswell and Arens, *The Role of Sanction in Conflict Resolution*, 11 J. OF CONFLICT RESOLUTION 27, (1967); Arens and Lasswell, *Toward A General Theory of Sanctions*, 49 IOWA L. REV. 233 (1964); R. ARENS AND H.D. LASSWELL, IN DEFENSE OF PUBLIC ORDER (1961).

[6] Durham v. United States, *supra* note 4.

[7] *Cf.*, e.g., Fisher v. United States, 328 U.S. 463 (1946) for a case reflective of the atmosphere of an earlier day.

[8] *See* e.g., Winn v. United States, 270 F.2d 326 (D.C. Cir 1959), Calloway v. United States, 270 F.2d 334 (D.C. Cir. 1959) which did indeed press the necessity of psychiatric examination to explore the feasibility of the insanity defense as a rule of law.

The verbal statement of the new rule of criminal responsibility required (if it was to be susceptible to implementation) a significant degree of public acceptance and the creation of material resources capable of making the goal of *treatment* rather than *punishment* a reality in an appreciable number of cases.[9]

In 1938 Professor George H. Dession warned:

> Any very extensive program of rehabilitation would require an assumption of responsibility of a degree to which our communities are unaccustomed.[10]

The primary question in any appraisal of such rule-making as is represented by *Durham* is the question of how far a given community is willing to assume meaningful responsibility for the acts of the mentally ill.

The District of Columbia scene (and one suspects that of many other jurisdictions) suggests that such willingness is diminutive.

THE COURT OF APPEALS AND A NEW RULE OF EXCULPATORY MENTAL ILLNESS

The Product Test

Exercising its right to frame a new standard of criminal responsibility,[11] the United States Court of Appeals for the District of Columbia had declared in *Durham v. United States*: "An accused is not criminally responsible if his un-

---

[9] *See* Dession, *Psychiatry and the Conditioning of Criminal Justice*, 47 YALE L.J. 319 (1938).

[10] *Id.* at 339.

[11] The United States Court of Appeals for the District of Columbia is entrusted with the formulation of a test of criminal responsibility to be applied in the District. Durham v. United States, 214 F.2d 862, 874 (D.C. Cir. 1954); Fisher v. .United States, 328 U.S. 463, 476-77 (1945).

lawful act was the product of mental disease or defect."[12]

Mental disease or defect remained undefined by the court beyond the statement that disease connoted "a condition which . . . [was] capable of either improving or deteriorat-

[12] Durham v. United States, *supra* at 874-75. In developing its basic theme the Court of Appeals further stated:
"The legal and moral traditions of the western world require that those who, of their own free will and with evil intent (sometimes called *mens rea*), commit acts which violate the law, shall be criminally responsible for those acts. Our traditions also require that where such acts stem from and are the product of a mental disease or defect as those terms are used herein, moral blame shall not attach, and hence there will not be criminal responsibility." *Id.* at 876.

As stated, the *Durham* rule does appear at first glance as "a peculiar mixture of Aristotelian Faculty Psychology, Metaphysics, Mysticism, and Medieval Theology." *See* Savage, *Discussion,* 116 AM. J. PSYCH. 295, 296 (1959).

Until the *Durham* case, the District of Columbia was governed by the *M'Naghten Rules* and the "irresistible impulse" test.

The *M'Naghten Rules* provided that it "must be clearly proved that, at the time of the committing of the act, the party accused was labouring under such a defect of reason, from disease of the mind, as not to know the nature and quality of the act he was doing; or if he did know it, that he did not know he was doing what was wrong." M'Naghten's case (1843), 8 E.R. 718. The *M'Naghten Rules* have been supplemented by the "irresistible impulse" test in the District of Columbia. That doctrine, as stated by the Court of Appeals, is that the degree of insanity which will relieve the accused of the consequences of a criminal act must be such as to create in his mind an uncontrollable impulse to commit the offense charged:

"This impulse must be such as to override the reason and judgment and obliterate the sense of right and wrong to the extent that the accused is deprived of the power to choose between right and wrong. . . . The accepted rule . . . is that the accused must be capable, not only of distinguishing between right and wrong, but that he was not impelled to do the act by an irresistible impulse, which means . . . that his reasoning powers were so far dethroned by his diseased mental condition as to deprive him of the will power to resist the insane impulse to perpetrate the deed, though knowing it to be wrong." Smith v. United States, 36 F.2d 548, 549 (D.C. Cir. 1929).

Significantly, upon the introduction of "some evidence of insanity the burden devolved upon the Government to prove sanity beyond reasonable doubt if it was to secure a conviction. *See* Davis v. United States, 160 U.S. 469 (1895). [All of this has now been purportedly changed by Nixonian legislation placing the burden of proof as to insanity on the defendant. *See* D.C. CODE §301 (j) (as amended in 1970).]

ing" and that defect connoted "a condition which [was] ... not considered capable of either improving or deteriorating."[13] The jury was thereafter no longer required to depend on artificial or arbitrarily selected symptoms derived from a more primitive age, but was to be guided instead by "wider horizons of knowledge."[14] As expressed by Judge Bazelon for the court:

> The question will be simply whether the accused acted because of a *mental disorder,* and not whether he displayed particular symptoms which medical science has long recognized do not necessarily, or even typically, accompany the most serious *mental disorder*.[15]

A flurry of litigation, much of it inspired by the architect of the *Durham* rule, followed what seemed at first glance a far-reaching and hopeful innovation in the courts.

The manifest content of *Durham* jurisprudence reflected a hodge-podge of purposes.[16] In the first flush of exuberance,

[13] Durham v. United States, *supra* at 876.
[14] *Id.* at 875. It is questionable whether the *Durham* rule, as thus stated, represents any significant innovation. Cognition need not be the only criterion of culpability under an enlightened interpretation of the rules of M'Naghten's case (1843), 8 E.R. 718.
See, *e.g.,* People v. Schmidt, 216 N.Y. 324, 110 N.E. 945 (1915); Stapleton v. The Queen, 86 Commw. L.R. 358 (Aug. 1, 1952). Dr. Frederic Wertham has made the point in these words:
"Judge Bazelon's . . . conclusion is . . . based on . . . psychiatric vagaries. . . . He substitutes a new test for the *M'Naghten* rules. In essence it requires that the plea of legal insanity must be based on a demonstration that the crime was the product of mental disease. If he had had better psychiatric advice, Judge Bazelon would have known that this is precisely how the *M'Naghten* rule has been interpreted in practice by experienced psychiatrists." Wertham, *Psychoauthoritarianism and the Law,* 22 U. Chi. L. Rev. 336 (1955).
For a more recent demonstration of the susceptibility of the M'Naghten Rules to enlightened psychiatric usage *see* F. Wertham, A Sign for Cain 229-86 (1966). These strictures however in no way detract from the humanitarian symbolism of the rule, and such symbolism surely cannot be a matter of indifference.
[15] Durham v. United States, *supra* at 876 (emphasis supplied).
[16] For a good description of evolving *Durham* doctrine *see* Krash, The *Durham Rule and Judicial Administration of the Insanity Defense in the District of Columbia,* 70 Yale L.J. 905 (1961).

Durham case law reflected the broadest possible expansion of the concept of exculpatory mental illness. The "right-wrong" test was viewed as inappropriate—at least as the sole determinant of criminal responsibility.[17] Reliance upon cognition was declared hazardous if not misleading. Traditional conceptions of insanity were derided as phrenological nonsense.[18] Impelled by "broader horizons of knowledge" the court later declared:

"The assumption that psychosis is a legally sufficient mental disease and that other illnesses are not is erroneous."[19]

When a juror, after several hours of deliberation "asked for further instructions as to whether 'in determining insanity . . . any other consideration . . . might be included . . . than dementia or schizophrenia,'" and the trial court refused to act upon his request, a conviction obtained in the case was reversed by the Court of Appeals.[20] As expressed by the Court of Appeals, "the refusal to answer the juror's question and the denial of the requested instruction constitute reversible error. . . ."[21]

The evolving *Durham* jurisprudence was of course subject to the gloss of constitutional and common law requirements as to "reasonable doubt" and burden of proof. Upon the presentation of "some evidence" of mental disease or defect "settled law . . . placed upon the prosecution the burden of proving sanity beyond a reasonable doubt."[22] In this context,

[17] See Durham v. United States, *supra* at 869-74.
[18] *Id.* at 867.
[19] Briscoe v. United States, 248 F.2d 640, 641 (D.C. Cir. 1957).
[20] Wright v. United States, 250 F.2d 4 (D.C. Cir. 1957).
[21] *Id.* at 11.
[22] Goforth v. United States, 269 F.2d 778, 779 (D.C. Cir. 1959) and *see* cases of Davis v. United States, 160 U.S. 469 (1895) *and* Tatum v. United States, 190 F.2d 612 (D.C. Cir. 1951) cited *therein*. But cf. the constitutionally dubious statutory provision of Nixonian vintage, placing the burden of proving the insanity defense on a defendant generally devoid of the requisite intellectual and financial resources for such a task. D.C. CODE §301(j) as amended 1970.

the burden of convincing the jury rested on the government. For it was the government which was then required to disprove either the defendant's pathological state or the existence of the necessary causal relationship and to do so beyond reasonable doubt. The nature of that burden was most aptly conveyed in negative terms. As expressed by the Court of Appeals, which disclaimed the formulation of "an instruction which would be either appropriate or binding in all cases," jury instructions under the *Durham* rule "should in some way convey to the jury the sense and substance of the following":

> If you, the jury, believe beyond a reasonable doubt that the accused was not *suffering* from a diseased or defective mental condition at the time he committed the criminal act charged, you may find him guilty. If you believe he was suffering from a diseased or defective mental condition when he committed that act, but believe beyond a reasonable doubt that the act was not the product of such mental abnormality, you may find him guilty. *Unless you believe beyond a reasonable doubt either that he was not suffering from a diseased or defective mental condition, or that the act was not the product of such abnormality, you must find the accused not guilty by reason of insanity.* Thus your task would not be completed upon finding, if you did find, that the accused suffered from a mental disease or defect. He would still be responsible for his unlawful act if there was no causal connection between such mental abnormality and the act. These questions must be determined by you from the facts which you find to be fairly deducible from the testimony and the evidence in this case.[23]

Criteria of Productivity

Dealing with the problem raised by the inherent ambiguity of what was or what was not a mental disease or defect productive of crime, the court declared that productivity need be judged solely in terms of a necessary or critical causal relationship between mental disease or defect on the one hand and criminal behavior on the other. This relation-

---

[23] Durham v. United States, *Supra* note 2, at 875 (emphasis supplied).

ship did not, as seen by the court, mean that the act under scrutiny must be "a direct emission, or a proximate creation, or an immediate issue of the disease," but rather that the "relationship between the disease and the act, ... *whatever it may be in degree*, ... be ... critical in respect to the act."[24]

Competency to Stand Trial

Competency to stand trial is in no way inconsistent with an insanity defense. An accused may be capable of rational and effective participation in his own defense and may still be able to raise the insanity defense as a victim of exculpatory mental illness. In other words, competency relates to present ability to withstand the stresses of the trial and participate in one's own defense; the assertion of the insanity defense relates to a past mental state. Under present law, a finding of competency may not be introduced by the prosecution as evidence of mental health to negative the defense of insanity.[25] Mental examinations to assess competency of an accused may fail to demonstrate a lack of competency to stand trial, but may in fact pinpoint exculpatory mental illness requiring an acquittal by reason of insanity.

The District of Columbia Code provided for mental examination at a government hospital upon a *prima facie* showing "that the accused is of unsound mind or ... mentally incompetent so as to be unable to understand the proceedings against him or to properly assist in his own defense...."[26] The Court of Appeals decided in 1959 that this statutory section was interpretable as authorizing or requir-

---

[24] Carter v. United States, 252 F.2d 608, 616, 617 (D.C. Cir. 1957) (emphasis supplied).

[25] *See* Lyles v. United States, 254 F.2d 725, 732 (D.C. Cir. 1957); Horton v. United States, 317 F.2d 595 (D.C. Cir. 1963).

[26] D.C. CODE ANN. §24-301(a), Supp. VIII, 1960. Cf. 18 U.S.C. §4244.

ing a mental examination on the issue of competency to stand trial as well as that on exculpatory mental illness.[27]

Significantly, the *Durham* court failed to provide concrete criteria as to competency to stand trial and has thus invited the conclusory statements of a public hospital that an accused was or was not competent.

One is further bound to observe that the concept of competency is dynamic and variable, deriving its meaning from the particular case situation from which it is drawn. A few illustrations should suffice.

An individual suffering from borderline mental deficiency may be competent to participate in his own defense where the charge involved is nothing more serious than simple assault. He is clearly not competent where the charge is one of financial fraud requiring a capacity to follow explanations of elaborate financial transactions. Such illustrations can be multiplied. Nothing in the jurisprudence of the Durham court suggests that competency is capable of gradations determined by the nature of the offense, the duration of the trial and the complexity of the testimony.[28]

It is worth noting too that the Supreme Court has moved far ahead of the Court of Appeals. Thus in *Dusky v. United States,* the Supreme Court declared more than one decade ago:

> It is not enough for . . . [a trial] judge to find that the defendant [is] oriented to time and place and [has] some recollection of events. . . . The test must be whether . . . (the defendant) has sufficient present ability to consult with his lawyer with a reasonable degree of rational understanding—and whether he has a rational as well as a factual understanding of the proceedings against him.[29]

More recently, the Supreme Court has held that a determination of competency could not be made mechanically and

---

[27] Winn v. United States, 270 F.2d 326 (D.C. Cir. 1959), Calloway v. United States, 270 F.2d 334 (D.C. Cir. 1959).
[28] *Cf.* Ross, *Commitment of the Mentally Ill: Problems of Law and Policy,* 57 MICH. L. REV. 945 (1959).
[29] Dusky v. United States, 362 U.S. 402 (1960).

that a "history of pronounced irrational behavior" could well outweigh an appearance of mental alertness and understanding in deciding upon the competency of the accused.[30] Only recently has the Court of Appeals attempted to inform both trial judges and psychiatrists that competency could not be judged by solely intellectual considerations. It has thus pointed out that such factors as pathological distrust of counsel might well be viewed as some evidence of incompetency.[31] As a practical matter, however, trial judges and psychiatrists in the District of Columbia have remained without guidelines as to the meaning of a matter essential to due process in criminal proceedings—the competency of the accused.

Model Testimony as Seen by the Court of Appeals

The Court of Appeals evinced a partiality toward what appeared to be a psychoanalytically-oriented account of human behavior. Label-pinning, suggestive of organic psychiatry, was to be avoided. As explained in *Carter v. United States*:[32]

[30] *See* Pate v. Robinson, 383 U.S. 349, 385-6 (1966).

[31] Pouncy v. United States, 375 F.2d 699 (D.C. Cir. 1965).

[32] Carter v. United States, *supra* at 617. Dr. Thomas Szasz observed that, absent a clear and objective finding of crime, not provided for under *Durham* jurisprudence as the explicit basis of psychiatric expert evidence, such "description and explanation" was not psychoanalytic but pseudo-psychoanalytic in character. He referred to Freud's strictures on the psychiatric mismanagement of testimony in the Halsman case. T. S. SZASZ, LAW, LIBERTY AND PSYCHIATRY 104-05 (1963). It must be observed in this connection, that the insanity defense in the District of Columbia may be postulated on a mere stipulation of the alleged criminal offense. *See also* United States v. Arduini, Criminal No. U.S. 10749-66 (D.C. Gen. Sess. 1967) for a judicial opinion affirmatively holding that acquittal on the basis of a reasonable doubt of mental illness was in no way inconsistent with the finding that a defendant at the time of a crime may "very well [have been] . . . without mental disease or mental disorder. . . ."

Description and explanation of the origin, development and manifestations of the alleged disease are the chief functions of the expert witness. The chief value of an expert's testimony in this field, as in all other fields, rests upon the material from which his opinion is fashioned and the reasoning by which he progresses from his material to his conclusion; in the explanation of the disease and its dynamics, that is, how it occurred, developed and affected the mental and emotional processes of the defendant....

The value of psychiatric testimony lay, in brief, in a mastery of the defendant's life history. Thus the court expressed its dissatisfaction with the quality of psychiatric testimony in the case of two defendants in these terms: "We know nothing of their childhood, their emotional states, the major events of their lives, their day-to-day behavior, their personalities, their own explanations for their behavior."[33]

Is a Right to Treatment a Corollary of the New Rule?

Notwithstanding the brave new insights of some of its opinions, the Court of Appeals intended to provide treatment for the beneficiary of the insanity defense exclusively upon an intramural basis and specifically within the confines of St. Elizabeths Hospital. It directed that the patient be detained until he had shed all manner of "abnormality" which suggested danger to society. In so doing it scrapped the rule enunciated by the Congress which permitted the detention of the patient only until such time as he had recovered his "sanity" and demonstrated his lack of dangerousness.[34]

[33] Rollerson v. United States, 343 F.2d 269, 272 (D.C. Cir. 1964).
[34] *See e.g.,* Overholser v. Russel, 283 F.2d 195 (D.C. Cir. 1960) which held that *bona fide* testimony by St. Elizabeths Hospital that an inmate had not fully recovered from a psychoneurotic check-writing proclivity was enough to bar release unless such testimony was disproved beyond reasonable doubt. In a word, the beneficiary of the insanity defense who sought release from St. Elizabeths Hospital had to meet draconian requirements fashioned by the Court of Appeals. He had to prove, beyond reasonable doubt, his freedom from "any abnormal condition" and that he was not likely to repeat the act which had resulted in his insanity acquittal. *See*
(Footnote continued on next page.)

One would assume that this draconian loss of liberty, defended in the name of "care and treatment," would be followed by continuing solicitude for "care and treatment" by the Court of Appeals. The attitude of the court, however, has been erratic, to say the least.

In 1962, the *Durham* court disclaimed any interest in existing treatment facilities at St. Elizabeths and asserted that the claim that the facilities at St. Elizabeths might not be as adequate as those furnished in a prison setting was without legal relevance.[35]

In 1966, in what appeared to be at first glance the pathbreaking case of *Rouse v. Cameron*, the court proclaimed a right to treatment for the St. Elizabeths patient, acquitted by reason of insanity, and declared that this particular right could be asserted by a *habeas corpus* petition.[36] When, however, in the same case upon remand, the District Court declared that the "milieu therapy" testified to by St. Elizabeths physicians in the District Court hearing was sufficient, the Court of Appeals chose to bypass every aspect of the

---

Arens, *Due Process and the Rights of the Mentally Ill: The Strange Case of Frederick Lynch,* 13 CATHOLIC U. L. REV. 22-25 (1964), *and* statutes and cases cited therein. In Bolton v. Harris, 395 F.2d 642 (D.C. Cir. 1968), the Court of Appeals held that an individual acquitted by reason of insanity was indeed subject to automatic commitment but solely to determine present illness or dangerousness. "The lengh of time required for . . . [necessary] examination [in the course of such commitment] will vary . . . with the individual case." The conclusion of the examination period was to be followed by a judicial hearing "similar to those in civil commitment proceedings." The hearing in turn was to determine whether further mental hospitalization was in order. *Ibid.* The case histories amassed by Dr. Thomas S. Szasz do not allow of a hopeful prognosis for a careful weighing of individual rights under such auspices. *See* T. S. SZASZ, LAW, LIBERTY AND PSYCHIATRY (1963) *and* T. S. SZASZ, PSYCHIATRIC JUSTICE (1965). *It is ironic that the Court which openly discouraged the assertion of an insanity defense founded on a nonpsychotic disorder since 1962, would nonetheless insist upon the civil commitability of nonpsychotic persons whose "mental illness" made them dangerous to themselves or others.* Bolton v. Harris, 395 F.2d 642 (D.C. Cir. 1968).
[35] Overholser v. O'Beirne, 302 F.2d 852, 854 (D.C. Cir. 1962).
[36] Rouse v. Cameron, 373 F.2d 451 (D.C. Cir. 1966).

treatment issue and decided the case upon other grounds.[37] A more dramatic illustration is provided by the case of an acutely psychotic young Negro whose extradition to North Carolina was sought in the District of Columbia. Notwithstanding uncontroverted psychiatric affidavits that treatment should precede extradition, and that extradition, without prior treatment would precipitate intensive suicidal attempts, the young Negro was shipped off to North Carolina on the strength of a Court of Appeals order. The order was joined in by Judge Bazelon.[38]

Early Repercussions in the District Court

Until 1962, early *Durham* jurisprudence was accompanied by a marked rise in insanity acquittals in the District of Columbia.[39] This was paralleled by an equally marked rise in requests for mental examinations—both to explore the relevancy of the insanity defense as well as to assess the competency of the individual defendant to stand trial.[40]

---

[37] *See* Rouse v. Cameron, 387 F.2d 241 (D.C. Cir. 1967). An appeal from the District Court's holdings was held moot on the assumption that the petitioner had filed another superseding *habeas corpus* petition. The latter had claimed illegal detention on the ground that the petitioner had not voluntarily asserted the insanity defense.

[38] *See* Lathan v. Reid, Clerk's File in the Court of Appeals case cited as 280 F.2d 66 (D.C. Cir. 1960) cert. den. 364 U.S. 865 (1960). The facts are available not only in the Clerk's file but also in the petition for *certiorari* in the Supreme Court. *See* Lathan v. Reid, No. 187 Misc. (D.C. Cir. 1960) cert. den. 364 U.S. 865 (1960). Significantly or otherwise the Court of Appeals' opinion made no reference to uncontroverted affidavits claiming that extradition was likely to trigger suicidal attempts. *See* Lathan v. Reid, 280 F.2d 66 (D.C. Cir. 1960).

[39] *See* A. Krash, *The Durham Rule and Judicial Administration of the Insanity Defense in the District of Columbia*, 70 YALE L. J. 905 (1961) *passim.*

[40] The Court of Appeals had assured defendants of the right to psychiatric examination on any reasonable grounds both for purposes of assessing competency to stand trial and exploring a possible insanity defense. *See* Winn v. United States, 270 F.2d 326 (D.C. Cir. 1959), Calloway v. United States, 270 F.2d 334 (D.C. Cir. 1959).

It is not unreasonable to assume that the psychiatric sophistication encountered among bench and bar in the District of Columbia was not easily matched by any other jurisdiction in the nation.

Judicial Retrenchment and Mental Disorder Under the New Rule

In the day to day administration of the insanity defense, the submerged content of *Durham* jurisprudence was in many ways more significant than what seemed manifest. What transpired was that a court, conspicuous for its sophistication in the understanding of psychodynamics, declined every invitation to pass upon the credibility of psychiatric testimony. As a practical matter this meant that the staff of St. Elizabeths, possessing, as it did, a virtual monopoly of critical mental examinations, had *carte blanche* in the determination of mental disease or defect and hence of criminal responsibility.[41] A classic illustration was provided by the situation in which St. Elizabeths psychiatrists testified that a narcotics addict of some twenty years standing was without mental disorder. When, upon argument in the Court of Appeals, the assertion was made that such testimony was as credible as the assertion that the earth was flat, the Court of Appeals held that a valid jury issue was presented; that is, that such testimony could be believed by reasonable men.[42] In drug addiction, as well as in other matters, the Court of Appeals would not interfere. Neither, it appears, would the American Psychiatric Association. A questionable latitude, moreover, was conceded by the Court of Appeals to

---

[41] One observes in passing that in the case of United States v. Vincent Gilleo, criminal case no. 583-59 (D.D.C. 1960), a Government psychiatrist declared with gay insouciance that it was his psychiatric opinion that the defendant was "criminally responsible."

[42] *See* Rivers case discussed *infra.* Ch. VII.

the trial courts which on occasion adopted a predominantly cognitive criterion in their jury charges.[43]

Inevitably the insanity defense of the District of Columbia became dependent, as suggested by Judge Irving Kaufman, on a psychiatric judgment which did not appear subject to any effective review.[44]

A mood of retrenchment dominated the Court of Appeals in the sixties.

While the court as a whole had, in the early phase of *Durham* jurisprudence, assented to the proposition that a nonpsychotic mental illness was sufficient for acquittal by reason of insanity,[45] it had at no time followed through by requiring the trial court to charge the jury to the same effect.

One is bound to note emphatically in this connection that a search of jury charges in the District Court of the District of Columbia covering the years 1959 through 1961 failed to disclose a single instance in which a jury had been explicitly apprised of the possibility of an acquittal founded on a finding of nonpsychotic mental disorder.

By the turn of the decade, the Court of Appeals was no longer referring to the insanity defense of the nonpsychotic individual as a desired end. A departure from the paths originally charted by *Durham* seemed at length to be dramatized in *McDonald v. United States*.[46] There, a panel of the court, including Judge Bazelon, the author of the *Durham* rule, held unanimously that acquittal by reason of insanity depended on a finding of such disease as "substantially affected mental or emotional processes and substantially impaired behavior controls."[47] As of 1963, the court seemed

---

[43] *See, e.g.,* Simpson v. United States, 320 F.2d 803 (D.C. Cir. 1963). *See also generally* Arens and Susman, *Judges, Jury Charges and Insanity,* 12 How. L. J. 1 (1966).
[44] United States v. Freeman, 357 F.2d 606, 621-22 (2d Cir. 1966).
[45] Briscoe v. United States, 248 F.2d 640 (D.C. Cir. 1957).
[46] 312 F.2d 847 (D.C. Cir. 1962).
[47] *Id.,* at 851.

explicitly bent upon repudiating the probability, if not the possibility, of an insanity acquittal based on nonpsychotic mental disorder. For it held:

> There must be a *serious* mental disease, and satisfactory evidence of causation, before a verdict of acquittal by reason of insanity must follow as a matter of law.[48]

By this time trial judges who sought to put "the right and wrong" gloss on the insanity charge could count on the support of a majority of the Court of Appeals Judges. By 1962, the wheel seemed to have turned full circle. In *Simpson v. United States,* decided in 1962, the Court of Appeals declined to find plain error in an insanity instruction by the District Court which read:

> As an example of this causal connection or relation, if a person at the time of the commission of a crime is so deranged mentally that he cannot distinguish between right and wrong, or, being able to tell right from wrong, he is unable by virtue of his mental derangement to control his actions, then his act is the product of his mental derangement.[49]

The observation does not seem inapposite that if the Court of Appeals had indeed sought to invite acquittal by reason of nonpsychotic mental disorder at any time, it was clearly no longer doing so by 1962 or thereafter.[50] The rate of insanity acquittals which had risen steadily since 1954

---

[48] Hightower v. United States, 325 F.2d 616, 619 (D.C. Cir. 1963) (emphasis supplied).

[49] 320 F.2d 803 (D.C. Cir. 1963).

[50] Nor does it seem inapposite to remark that where the issue before the court was release from confinement at St. Elizabeths Hospital as distinct from hospitalization as an alternative to imprisonment in the conventional sense, the court continued to recognize the broadest spectrum of nonpsychotic psychopathology—significantly as a basis for the denial of liberty. *See e.g.,* Overholser v. Leach, 257 F.2d 667 (D.C. Cir. 1958); Overholser v. Russell, 283 F.2d 195 (D.C. Cir. 1960) and *see* ARENS, *Due Process and the Rights of the Mentally Ill: The Strange Case of Frederick Lynch,* 13 CATHOLIC U.L. REV. 3 (1964) Cf. Bolton v. Harris, 395 F.2d (D.C. Cir. 1968).

through 1962 registered a marked decline after these cases. Proof is found in the following table:

PERSONS FOUND NOT GUILTY BY REASON OF INSANITY
(U. S. District Court for the District of Columbia, fiscal years 1954-1966)

Fiscal Year	Defendants in Cases Terminated*	Defendants in Cases Tried*	Defendants NGI-	NGI as Percent of Defendants in Cases Terminated	NGI as Percent of Defendants in Cases Tried
1954★	1,870	673	3	0.2	0.4
1955	1,384	453	8	.6	1.8
1956	1,595	456	16	1.0	3.5
1957	1,454	456	7	.5	1.5
1958	1,666	522	17	1.0	3.3
1959	1,642	528	32	1.9	6.1
1960	1,367	400	35	2.6	8.8
1961	1,337	457	66	4.9	14.4
1962	1,282	480	66	5.1	13.8
1963	1,183	398	53	4.5	13.3
1964	1,142	393	23	2.0	5.9
1965	1,286	372	35	2.7	9.4
1966	1,230	380	26	2.1	6.8
Total	18,438	5,968	387	2.1	6.5

*Source: Administrative Office of the United States Courts. [Abstracted from President's Commission on Crime in the District of Columbia, Report 535 (1966) —ed.]
- "NGI" = not guilty by reason of insanity in this and subsequent tables.
★ The fiscal year preceding the decision in *Durham* v. *United States*. Prior to this year, insanity patients were not recorded separately from all other prisoner patients at Saint Elizabeths Hospital.

Nonetheless, the *Durham* court persisted in lip service to classic concepts of earlier *Durham* jurisprudence, sometimes declaring that the *McDonald* case, to take that example, was illustrative of the continuing solicitude of the court for an insanity defense consistent with "wider horizons of knowledge."[51]

---

[51] The expression "wider horizons of knowledge" is, of course, embodied in Durham v. United States, 214 F.2d 862, 875 (D.C. Cir. 1954).
(Footnote continued on next page.)

In this process the court effected, if not an expanded insanity defense, a not insignificant "credibility gap" between itself and the students of its decisions.

A recent case in which *McDonald* was deemed consistent with early Durham jurisprudence was Washington v. United States, 380 F.2d 444 (D.C. Cir. 1967). The majority of judges in that case declared that it was the view of the Court that "psychiatrists . . . [are] prohibited from testifying whether the alleged offense was the 'product' of mental illness since this . . . [was] part of the ultimate issue to be decided by the jury." *Id.* at 455. Significantly, however, since the conviction obtained below was affirmed, the language of the Court of Appeals in this matter must be viewed as mere *dictum*.

Chapter II

A SHORT HISTORY OF A PROJECT IN INSANITY RESEARCH AND LITIGATION

A PROJECT IS BORN

Still in 1959, and before this avalanche, the Norman Foundation of New York made a grant to the Washington School of Psychiatry to study the development of the insanity defense in the District of Columbia. I became director of the project. An advisory board was established under the auspices of the Washington School. It included a member of the United States Court of Appeals for the District of Columbia. Intermittent contact was maintained between the advisory board and the project staff over a period of several years.

The initial question—restated in over-simplified form for the project staff—was what practical meaning was to be attached to what some people had regarded as a revolutionary innovation on the Anglo-American legal scene.

My major interest was the testing of the hypothesis, advanced by the United States Court of Appeals for the District of Columbia Circuit in an opinion written by Judge Bazelon, that *"the assumption that psychosis . . . [was] a legally sufficient mental disease and that other illnesses . . . [were not] . . . was erroneous."*[1]

Initial research focused upon the overt attitudes expressed by private psychiatrists as to their role in criminal courtroom work with a view to sifting dominant attitudes.

---

[1] Briscoe v. United States, 248 F.2d 640, 641 (D.C. Cir. 1957).

Results of the interviews of private and public psychiatrists conducted by the project produced superficial results.

Thirty-five interviews were conducted *in toto* by project staff members. The evasive nature of the psychiatric response permitted only impressionistic analysis. Understanding of the legal doctrine among those psychiatrists appeared haphazard. Little systematic thinking seemed reflected in answers to questions posed by interviewers as to the nature of exculpatory mental illness. All of the psychiatrists had been selected because of their frequency of criminal courtroom work. All but four of them thought that the law required an illness of psychotic or near-psychotic proportions to justify an insanity defense.

All but three psychiatrists admitted being influenced by a whole complex of extra-medical considerations in the expressions of their diagnostic viewpoints. Some seemed barely conscious of what they were about. Others had a clear-cut awareness of the impact of such extra-medical considerations and made their admissions with varying degrees of self-assurance or embarrassment. Those possessed of sufficient awareness often labored under the distinct impression that the duty of legal, social, economic and metaphysical analysis devolved upon them alongside the more routine duties of making medical diagnoses in cases involving criminal responsibility.

Those whose extra-medical excursions caused embarrassment seemed best represented by a nationally prominent Baltimore psychoanalyst. When I contacted him by telephone to inquire as to his views on chronic narcotics addiction, I was emphatically informed that he regarded addiction as symptomatic of a severe mental disorder. When queried as to whether he was willing to express this view in the course of District Court proceedings in a criminal trial, he inquired as to whether an insanity defense was being propounded. When I replied that it was, he proceeded to raise such highly relevant questions from the standpoint of the social disposition of narcotic delinquents as the present availability of hospital space and therapeutic facilities which might make an insanity defense at that particular time meaningful. His discussion of the social implications of the psychiatric approach to the narcotics delinquent in the courtroom waxed so eloquent and the expression of his doubts concerning the wisdom of an insanity defense so great that I felt constrained to remind him that while I shared much of his own concern in several of these matters, I had consulted him solely with a view to securing his medical, not his socioeconomic views upon the subject. He replied with the instant reaffirmation of his earlier thesis as to the nature of narcotics addiction but declined to say whether he would testify in that case until he had time for further reflection. Further reflection resulted in his refusal to testify.

Interviews with some five senior staff members at St. Elizabeths Hospital—including medical staff members of the hospital administration—left an even stronger impression of extra-diagnostic judgments in the handling of criminal cases processed through the hospital. All but one of these physicians made the point that they regarded criminality as not an illness but "a way of life." All asserted that they were unable to ignore the impact of the housing shortage on decision-making in this context.

Highlights of some of these interviews deserve reproduction.

When asked whether he was influenced in his decisions by the impact that his decisions would exert upon the courtroom process and the ultimate finding of guilt or innocence, Dr. X of St. Elizabeths Hospital replied in the affirmative. He added spontaneously that he was "also influenced by the impact that his decision would exert upon St. Elizabeths Hospital in terms of housing."

Asked at the outset of the interview as to whether he accepted the *American Psychiatric Association Diagnostic and Statistical Manual* as a valid classification of mental disorders, a medical administrator at St. Elizabeths Hospital replied that as far as his personal opinion was concerned he did not. He then went on to say:

> I am not convinced that all crime is the result of psychiatric conditions. It is not practical to look at it that way. I am concerned with those who can benefit from the treatment facilities at St. Elizabeths Hospital.

Twenty-seven criminal defense lawyers selected essentially upon the basis of a heavy criminal case load were also interviewed. All but a handful appeared cognition-oriented. The handful, significantly, appeared to have total understanding and sympathy for what appeared to be the Court of Appeals' view in early *Durham* jurisprudence. All but one of the defense lawyers interviewed expressed the view that District Court judges tended to view the insanity defense with suspicion and at times hostility.

An attempt to interview members of the United States Attorney's office turned out to be unsuccessful. The senior and presumably policy-making members of the organization flatly refused to be interviewed. Several junior members who agreed to interviews were unable or unwilling to discuss the dynamics of critical decision-making by their office touching the insanity defense.

THE PROJECT EXPANDS TO INCLUDE INSANITY DEFENSE LITIGATION

Still under the auspices of the Washington School of Psychiatry, I applied for a grant which would permit greater depth in the appraisal of the psychiatric defense in the District Court within the District of Columbia. My feeling was that not only psychiatrists but judges and jurors as well needed to be studied, and studied as intensively as circumstances would permit within the context of actual and live trials of criminal cases in which an insanity defense was interposed. In brief, the project which in 1961 secured a subsidy from the National Institute of Mental Health (N.I.H.) sought to address itself to the task of actual litigation involving the insanity defense in which the cases selected whenever possible, involve[d] psychopathology of the *nonpsychotic* type and the defense could rationally and legally be based on a liberal interpretation of the local rule of criminal responsibility.[2]

The inquiry was to be addressed to the issue of whether the "wild beast" test or the rigid version of nineteenth century interpretations of *M'Naghten* had in fact been scrapped, or whether they continued to assert significant influence upon key decision-makers.

The major context of data gathering was to be that of the live trial in which the key issue was the defense of insanity. This was to be done under the direct and immediate supervision of the project director.

In the application to the National Institute of Mental Health it was made clear that in any conflict between the interest of scientific or legal investigation and that of a defendant in a criminal case, it was the interest of scientific or legal investigation which would be sacrificed. For example, notwithstanding the belief of a responsible trial lawyer in charge of a project case that a given individual was a victim of a minor mental illness which could be meaningfully related to his crime by appropriate psychiatric testimony under the *Durham* rule and that the exploration of such a procedure was both scientifically and legally justifiable, the wishes of a defendant would be viewed as decisive in shaping the final decision as to whether an insanity defense was or was not to be propounded.

Other data-gathering instruments proposed and accepted by the National Institute of Mental Health included content analysis of judicial instructions to the jury in cases in which the insanity defense had been raised, and interviews of such prime decision-makers as jurors and psychiatrists.

---

[2] N.I.H. Research Plan M. 5009.

The grant provided by the National Institute of Mental Health set aside substantial funds for the utilization of private psychiatrists in court cases in which the opposition of psychiatrists secured by the government would seem to render the insanity defense illusory, unless the defense secured psychiatrists of its own.

The arrangement by which cases were obtained was a straightforward one. The Legal Aid Office in the District Court was informed that project staff members were available to take charge of indigent cases in criminal court, regardless of whether or not the cases involved the probable assertion of the insanity defense. Several cases tried by the project did not involve any phase of the insanity defense. The Clerk's Office of the District Court was likewise informed. Both cooperated handsomely until stopped by the District Court.

More than twenty cases were tried both by the project director and his staff. An uncounted number of cases benefited from the psychiatric expertise furnished by the project to lawyers bereft of adequate psychiatric facilities.

The trial case did indeed live up to all of one's expectations and in fact provided *data* which seemed unexpected at the time when project operations began.

OPPOSITION TO THE PROJECT GATHERS MOMENTUM

Initial opposition to the project was haphazard and superficial. Members of the United States Attorney's office refused to be interviewed. Psychiatrists—both in private practice and at St. Elizabeths Hospital—were evasive in many instances. An occasional project-retained psychiatrist would be cross-examined with special vigor by a member of the prosecuting staff as to his affiliation with the project. After the 1961 subsidy from the National Institute of Mental Health, overt resistance to the project took approximately one year to materialize. The first storm signals appeared in the conduct of jury interviews. Initially authorized by the bench, the commencement of interviews of jurors who had completed their jury service resulted almost instantaneously in charges made by two District Court judges that this practice involved an unjustifiable intrusion into, if not an actual subversion of, the court system. A more serious charge leveled against both the director and his staff was that of *champerty, barratry* and *maintenance* as well as an undefined conflict of interests. One notes in passing that similar charges, clearly designed to inhibit legal aid to the poor on a group basis, albeit financed by the Government itself, have since led to similar reactions, and that appellate courts have judged them to be without merit.[3] Several members of the United States Attorney's office rose in open court to announce that project counsel had succeeded in pushing himself into a given case in violation of professional canons of ethics.

The inevitable attack upon the wholesale failure of public psychiatric facilities and personnel to meet the needs of the new rule resulted not only in attacks upon the project director, highlighted by a formal charge of intimidation, but in a large scale joinder in that attack by leading members of the private psychiatric profession in the District of Columbia who rushed to the support of St. Elizabeths Hospital.

In the case of *United States v. Kent,* the intimation made directly from the bench was that intrusion into the case of an indigent defendant of psychiatrists paid from Government or private sources constituted a "synthetic activity and if this was so, somebody was going to get into serious trouble."[4] A hearing, ordered by the Court of Appeals, as to the propriety of Juvenile Court action in "waiving" jurisdiction and transferring the case of a sixteen year old boy for

[3] *See e.g.,* N.A.A.C.P. v. Buttons, 371 U.S. 415 (1963), Touchy v. Houston Legal Foundation Texas, 417 S.W. 2d 65, (1967).

[4] Proceedings before Chief Judge McGuire, Feb. 18, 1963, United States v. Kent (D.D.C. 1963).

trial by an adult court on capital charges was turned by the District Court into a hearing on the nefarious role of the director and his project and the *éminence grise* represented by the Washington School of Psychiatry, which—in the view of some of the judges and prosecutors—had committed the unpardonable crime: that of furnishing psychiatric witnesses without cost to indigent defendants.[5]

THE PROJECT DIES

Cases were denied to the project from there on in, and in fact some time before then. Word was passed to the Clerk's Office, the Assignment Office and the Legal Aid Office in the District Court that no cases were thereafter to be handed to the project staff. Several members of the Bar quoted two judges as stating that the matter would be taken further, and indeed it was. A formal opinion was sought from the Comptroller General of the United States as to the fundamental legality of the project. A formal opinion by the Comptroller General was in fact handed down. It absolved the project of dishonesty, but declared the litigative phase of the project to be improper and denied any further disbursement of funds for the financing of litigation.[6] It asserted that the use of public funds for study of the insanity defense by litigation was outside the bounds of Congressional authorization, and it pointed with apparent consternation at the disproportion of defense to government psychiatrists in one of the cases handled under project auspices. The decision was accepted without protest by the project's advisory board.

Not the solitary Purple Heart claimed for the University of Chicago in its jury study,[7] but a series of such Purple

[5] Kent v. United States, 383 U.S. 541 (1966) (Record before the Supreme Court.)
[6] *See* Appendix I
[7] *See* H. KALVEN, JR. & H. ZEISEL, THE AMERICAN JURY VII (1966).

Hearts (which failed to result in chronic incapacitation), rendered operations difficult and at times impossible. It is with a feeling of some pride, therefore, that one recalls the project as having succeeded in raising to the level of Supreme Court scrutiny the deprivational aspects of two cases involving the application of mental health and juvenile sanctions or sanction-equivalents. In the *Lynch* case[8] the Supreme Court held the automatic commitment clause of the District of Columbia law to be inapplicable to the case of an individual who had not voluntarily asserted the insanity defense on his own behalf; in the *Kent* case[9] the Supreme Court held that Juvenile Court proceedings determinative of whether the case of a child was to be "waived" or transferred to an adult court required assistance of counsel and comprehended the right to scrutiny of the once-secret social service dossier.[10] The case, in fact, broke the ice and led almost immediately to a Supreme Court holding that a child, no less than an adult, was entitled to effective assistance of counsel in every sense in a case in which Juvenile Court jurisdiction had in fact been assumed and exercised.[11] *Lynch* and *Kent* were both project cases.

---

[8] Lynch v. Overholser, 369 U.S. 705 (1962).
[9] Kent v. United States, 383 U.S. 541 (1966).
[10] *Ibid*.
[11] Application of Gault, 387 U.S. 1 (1967). (This was not a project case).

CHAPTER III

JUDICIAL PSYCHIATRY AND PSYCHIATRIC JUSTICE

Impressions gleaned from a study of the preceding require further validation through the scrutiny of what appears to be the major problem area: judicial psychiatry and psychiatric justice. What are the generalizations that one may permit oneself in describing the more or less consistent attitudes and practices of judges and psychiatrists who deal with the mentally or emotionally disturbed offender in the District of Columbia?

THE DURHAM COURT

Durham jurisprudence began with a sonorous disclaimer of cognition as the exclusive criterion of criminal responsibility. Years have passed. It is ironic that the tolerance of *Durham* jurisprudence for intellectual awareness as a criterion of criminal responsibility should have exceeded that of enlightened interpretations of *M'Naghten*.[1]

And indeed judicial psychiatry in the District of Columbia has been and continues to be passing strange.

The court's support of the widest possible spectrum of

---

[1] *See* Arens and Susman, *Judges, Jury Charges and Insanity*, 12 How. L.J. 1 (1966) and the cases cited therein. *Cf.* People v. Schmidt, 216 N.Y. 324, 110 N.E. 945 (1915); Stapleton v. The Queen, 86 COMMW. L.R. 358 (Aug. 1, 1952); Wertham, *Psychoauthoritarianism and the Law*, 22 U. CHI. L. REV. 336 (1955); *and* F. WERTHAM, A SIGN FOR CAIN 229-86 (1966).

exculpatory mental illnesses, consistent with accepted psychiatric usage, has withered on affirmances of convictions resting on the testimony of St. Elizabeths physicians that drug addicts, epileptics, sex perverts and victims of delusionary and hallucinatory experiences are without mental disease or defect.[2]

The grotesque posture of present appellate doctrine is best appreciated by juxtaposing the rules governing chronic alcoholics and drug addicts respectively. Chronic alcoholics have thus been declared to be victims of an illness and hence held immune from prosecution for the manifestation of such symptoms of their illness as public drunkenness.[3] In contrast, the chronic drug addict may (if described as "without mental disorder" by the St. Elizabeths staff) —be subject to the rigorous terms of imprisonment provided for under the Narcotics Statutes.[4]

The court, too, continued to prescribe treatment for the beneficiary of the insanity defense regardless of the nature of his mental disorder in a mental hospital "designed principally for the treatment of persons suffering from acute and chronic psychosis."[5]

[2] The doctrine of "inherent implausibility" often invoked against complaining witnesses in rape cases, did not seem to be applied to St. Elizabeths physicians on judicial review. *See e.g.,* State v. Morrison, 189 Iowa 1027, 179 N.W. 321 (1920); Brown v. Commonwealth, 82 Va. 653 (1886); *Cf.* People v. Carey, 223 N.Y. 519, 119 N.E. 83 (1918). *See also generally* J. MILLER, CRIMINAL LAW 294 (1934).

[3] *See* Easter v. United States, 361 F.2d 50 (D.C. Cir. 1966).

[4] *See* 26 U.S.C. §4704a; 26 U.S.C. §4742 (1956); 26 U.S.C. §4704 (a) (1954); 26 U.S.C. §4744 (a) (1956), *and* THE PRESIDENT'S ADVISORY COMMISSION ON NARCOTIC AND DRUG ABUSE, *Final Report* 40 (1963). *See* Appendix III for more recent citations.

[5] The description of St. Elizabeths Hospital as a hospital "designed principally for the treatment of persons suffering from acute and chronic psychoses" is that of Dr. Mauris Platkin, one of St. Elizabeths senior psychiatric physicians. *See Platkin, A Decade of Durham,* 32 MEDICAL ANNALS OF THE DISTRICT OF COLUMBIA 317, 318 (1963) also referred to *infra*. The rigidity with which institutionalization is prescribed by the court within a setting "designed principally for the treatment of persons suffering from acute and chronic psychoses" is best borne out by Overholser v. Russell, 283 F.2d 195 (D.C. Cir. 1960).

(Footnote continued on next page.)

As previously noted, the concern of the court for adequacy of treatment facilities was at best haphazard. The refusal of the court to analyze the merits of the testimonial assertions of St. Elizabeths Hospital as to the mental health of the epileptic, the drug addict, the sex pervert and the victim of delusionary and hallucinatory experiences, did not bespeak a significant concern for the victim of mental disease or defect.

PSYCHIATRIC JUSTICE

An assay of public psychiatry in the District of Columbia, undertaken by the project, alongside of the study of the attitudes manifested by trial judges and juries, found the psychiatric opposition to an expanding insanity defense no whit less than that of the psychiatrically unsophisticated public. Psychiatric attitudes, particularly those encountered at St. Elizabeths Hospital, were marked by massive fears of the breakdown of the already scarce resources of the public hospital and by the unexpectedly punitive orientation of public psychiatrists.

What were the constraints which the social structure of St. Elizabeths exercised on the administration of the *Durham* rule? What, moreover, was the character of that administration? For answers, we must turn to an examination of the available human and material resources and their use.

A relaxation of this rule is highlighted—at least upon a doctrinal plane—by Bolton v. Harris, 395 F.2d 642 (D.C. Cir. 1968). Under the Bolton rule, automatic commitment is still possible following the successful assertion of an insanity defense, but for observation only. Thereafter, continued confinement requires a court order based upon a hearing. This writer is frankly skeptical as to the likelihood that this innovation will produce any significant improvement in the picture.

POOR MAN'S PSYCHIATRY
AND ST. ELIZABETHS HOSPITAL

Facilities

The poor of Washington depend on public psychiatric facilities for exploration of such questions as competency to stand trial and responsibility as affected by mental disease or defect.

Almost invariably an order for a mental examination entered by the District Court commits the criminal defendant to the diagnostic care and custody of St. Elizabeths Hospital. Even in the rare case in which the defendant has sufficient means to secure independent psychiatric examination, an order for his examination by the St. Elizabeths staff will usually be entered by the court, and the defendant may be explicitly directed to cooperate with the St. Elizabeths physicians with the intimation that his lawyers may be cited for contempt if he does not.

Thus, St. Elizabeths is, in all but the rarest of cases, the ultimate arbiter of the existence of mental disease or defect for the people of the District of Columbia.

Home to approximately 7,000 mental patients, St. Elizabeths is conspicuously understaffed and overcrowded. As described by one of its senior physicians, it was "designed principally for the treatment of persons suffering from acute and chronic psychosis."[6] It is in no way atypical of public mental institutions elsewhere which have been described as "unmanageably large . . . , economically depressed, running on a fraction of the costs of general hospitals, schools or jails, . . . chronically understaffed, and . . . usually cut off from the main stream of professional life."[7]

---

[6] Platkin, *A Decade of Durham,* 32 MEDICAL ANNALS OF THE DISTRICT OF COLUMBIA 317, 318 (1963).

[7] Cumming and Cumming, *Social Equilibrium and Social Change in the Large Mental Hospital;* M. Greenblatt, D. Levinson & R. Williams, *The Patient and the Mental Hospital* 49 (1957).

The minimal budgetary allocation St. Elizabeths receives per patient per day bespeaks the scarcity of its resources and rules out any meaningful attempt at individualized treatment. Total costs per patient per day have been reported as $8.88 for the fiscal year of 1962, $10.30 for the fiscal year 1963, and $11.22 for the fiscal year of 1964. Of those costs, allocation for food per patient per day was 84 cents for the fiscal year of 1962, and 93 cents for the fiscal years 1963 and 1964, respectively.[8]

[8] Another dimension is obtained by examining a summary of total annual budgetary authorizations for St. Elizabeths Hospital for the period of 1957 to 1967 which was forwarded to Dr. Robert G. Kvarnes of the Washington School of Psychiatry on April 13, 1967. The figures reflect some rise in appropriations for St. Elizabeths. Nothing in these figures, however, suggests the wholesale reorientation of the hospital to accommodate the vast numbers of non-psychotic as well as psychotic patients eligible for insanity acquittals at least until MacDonald v. United States, 312 F. 2d 847 (D.C. Cir. 1962).

DEPARTMENT OF HEALTH, EDUCATION, AND WELFARE
SAINT ELIZABETHS HOSPITAL
History of Authorizations
1957-1967

Fiscal Year	Salaries and Expenses Appropriation Direct Appropriations	Reimbursements	Total Program	Buildings and Facilities Appropriations	Total for Hospital
1957	$2,870,000	$11,886,782	$14,756,782	$7,764,000	$22,520,782
1958	3,165,800	12,857,801	16,023,601	235,000	16,258,601
1959	3,442,000	13,674,285	17,116,285	212,000	17,328,285
1960	3,805,000	14,682,725	18,487,725	330,000	18,817,725
1961	4,572,000	16,285,415	20,857,415	5,445,000	26,302,415
1962	5,105,000	17,392,801	22,497,801	645,209	23,143,010
1963	6,332,000	19,623,576	25,955,576	8,095,000	34,050,576
1964	7,852,172	20,056,828	27,909,000	627,000	28,536,000
1965	9,619,897	19,749,103	29,369,000	2,032,000	31,401,000
1966	10,289,591	20,323,409	30,613,000	1,977,000	32,590,000
1967	8,865,000[a]	22,693,000[a]	31,558,000	2,298,000	33,856,000
1967 Suppl.[b]	995,000	52,000	1,047,000	—	1,047,000

a Starting with 1954, the Hospital began operating with an indefinite appropriation, under which it receives, in appropriated funds, the difference between reimbursements and its total authorized operating program. Accordingly, the direct appropriation and reimbursement figures shown for 1967 should be regarded as estimates.

b Proposed supplemental appropriation to cover general schedule and wage board salary increases.

It is inevitable under these circumstances that St. Elizabeths should be incapable of meeting the standards of the American Psychiatric Association for public mental hospitals. It must be recalled in this connection that "these standards represent a compromise between what was thought to be adequate and what it was thought had some *possibility* of being realized."[9] One encounters cases in which a patient is placed in a ward housing 1,000 patients and which provides two psychiatrists for their care and treatment.[10]

Contact with the hospital by the Project over a period of four years has confirmed the impression of others that as

> in many [other] mental hospitals there is a record [at St. Elizabeths] of disgruntled psychiatrists asserting they are leaving so they can do psychotherapy. Often a special psychiatric service, such as group psychotherapy, psychodrama or art therapy, is introduced with great support from high hospital management; then slowly interest is transferred elsewhere and the professional in charge finds that gradually his job has been changed into a species of public relations work—his therapy given only token support except when visitors come to the institution and high management is concerned to show how modern and complete the facilities are.[11]

If the *Durham* court had intended the accommodation of a significant number of nonpsychotic patients on the premises of St. Elizabeths Hospital after an insanity acquittal, it had not made—and it is not likely it had the power to make—any effective provision for their care.[12] It is clear, too, that Congress had not made a budgetary increase sufficient to permit accommodation of any significant number of nonpsychotic patients. In the halcyon year of 1957, the

---

[9] Solomon, *The American Psychiatric Association in Relation to American Psychiatry*, 115 AM. J. PSYCHIATRY 1, 7 (1958); for the standards themselves *see* AMERICAN PSYCHIATRIC ASSOCIATION STANDARDS FOR HOSPITALS AND CLINICS, 44-45 (1958).
[10] Lynch v. Overholser, Habeas Corpus No. 171-60 (1960).
[11] E. GOFFMAN, ASYLUMS 92 (1961).
[12] Overholser v. O'Beirne, 302 F.2d 852 (D.C. Cir. 1962).

court declared that "the assumption that psychosis is a legally sufficient mental disease and that other illnesses are not, . . . [was] erroneous."[13] Since that time, congressional appropriations for St. Elizabeths have not been such as to suggest inclusion within the Hospital of a large number of offenders who could be regarded as victims of a nonpsychotic mental disorder. It should be recalled in this connection that the incidence of moderate through severe symptom formation in a sampling of 1,660 midtown adults in a metropolitan community has been found to be 42.5 per cent.[14] The rise in appropriations—considering the increase in the cost of living—cannot, by any stretch of the imagination, be viewed as capable of encompassing a modest fraction of the influx suggested by such figures.

Overcrowding and understaffing give rise to such anomalies as confinement of a nonpsychotic alcoholic in a locked ward with acutely psychotic patients. Although unabated, such a practice gives rise to occasional expressions of indignation by the courts. In one case for example, a District Court judge declared:

> It may be that this petitioner needs hospitalization. Obviously, she should not be among insane people. There was a time when in-

---

[13] Briscos v. United States, 248 F.2d 640, 641 n.2 (D.C. Cir 1957).

[14] L. SROLE et al., MENTAL HEALTH IN THE METROPOLIS [The Mid-Town Manhattan Study].

T.A.C. RENNIE SERIES IN SOCIAL PSYCHIATRY (1962) reports as follows with regard to a sample of 1,660 mid-town adults:

Table 8-3. Home Survey Sample (Age 20-59), Respondents' Distribution on Symptom-formation Classification of Mental Health

Well	18.5%	
Mild symptom formation	36.3%	
Moderate symptom formation	21.8%	
Marked symptom formation	13.2%	
Severe symptom formation	7.5%	
Incapacitated	2.7%	
Impaired*		23.4%
N = 100%	(1,660)	

* Marked, Severe, and Incapacitated combined.

Id. at 138.

sane people were placed in jails, temporarily at least. We looked at this as a barbaric custom that has been pretty well eliminated. But we have reverted to it in reverse, we are placing sane people in insane institutions, which I think is even more barbaric. [15]

In the light of existing resources and the rigorous release procedures enforced by the District of Columbia courts, the plight of many a patient, acquitted by reason of insanity, and confined to St. Elizabeths Hospital, including the victim of the nonpsychotic disorder, is all too frequently the plight of a prisoner without hope of release.

One such prisoner, who sought his release upon *habeas corpus* after acquittal by reason of insanity, provided the following uncontradicted testimony as to lack of treatment at St. Elizabeths Hospital in his *habeas corpus* hearing:

THE DEFENSE: Mr. Pettit, where do you reside?

THE WITNESS: Right now at St. Elizabeths Hospital, John Howard Pavilion.

THE DEFENSE: How long have you been in St. Elizabeths Hospital at John Howard Pavilion?

THE WITNESS: I have been back there six months and four days.

THE DEFENSE: Mr. Pettit, would you tell the Court what your average day at the John Howard Pavilion is? . . .

THE WITNESS: In the mornings, after the breakfast meal, average day is about—helping clean up the ward, and I am chairman of the ward committee there and I check around and make sure everyone is helping to clean up, and I take care of my personal needs, maybe write a letter or something like that. Other times I practice a little bit on a musical instrument I play.

In the afternoons, I usually go to the John Howard Journal, where I work as a clerk. It's, you know,

---

[15] Tremblay v. Overholser, Habeas Corpus No. 288-1961 (D.D.C. 1961), *also cited* as 199 F. Supp. 569 (D.D.C. 1961).

voluntary services, and I go up and type to help, you know, make the paper, to put the John Howard paper out.

THE DEFENSE: What do you do after that?

THE WITNESS: Well, in the evening there is nothing more to do except watch television or write letters, read a book, and that's all there is.

. . . .

THE DEFENSE: And is this how you spend your days?

THE WITNESS: Yes, sir.

THE DEFENSE: Mr. Pettit, are you receiving any individual or group psychotherapy?

THE WITNESS: No, sir.

THE DEFENSE: Are you receiving any medication, Mr. Pettit?

THE WITNESS: No, sir.

THE DEFENSE: Are you receiving any vocational training, guidance, or counseling designed to fit you for a lawful life in free society?

THE WITNESS: No, sir. The only thing that is happening to me there that I can see is I am being held a prisoner there.[16]

After the discharge of his writ and during the pendency of his appeal, Pettit escaped from St. Elizabeths Hospital. He has not been heard from since.

Dr. Thomas Szasz, in commenting upon a comparable situation, observed:

> Mental hospitalization of this kind reminds one of the tales of the Count of Monte Cristo that is, of indefinite detention in jails without possibilities of legal reprieve, intelligently conceived and skillfully executed escape being the only means for gaining one's freedom. [17]

---

[16] Pettit v. Overholser, U.S.C.A., No. 16, 792, J.A. at 11-12 (D.C. Cir. 1961).

[17] Szasz, *Hospital Refusal to Release Mental Patient*, 9 CLEV. MAR. L. REV. 220, 223-24 (1960).

The atmosphere engendered by such conditions is not conducive to hope among incarcerated patients.

Designed "principally for the treatment of persons suffering from acute and chronic psychosis," St. Elizabeths Hospital clearly has not received sufficient funds to reconstitute itself as a treatment center for psychoneuroses and personality disorders as well.[18]

Social Structure and Ideology

The authoritarian atmosphere at St. Elizabeths Hospital appeared to be consistent with recent research on the public

---

[18] The attitude of the Court of Appeals toward a constitutional right of adequate and humane treatment of those confined within St. Elizabeths Hospital has varied through a period of approximately two decades.

An early concern for the fate of those confined within St. Elizabeths Hospital was replaced by apparent callousness. *Compare* Miller v. Overholser, 206 F.2d 415 (D.C. Cir. 1953) *with* Overholser v. O'Beirne, 302 F.2d 852, 854 (D.C. Cir. 1962).

In what appeared at first glance as a path breaking decision in 1966 the Court of Appeals declared that there was a right to treatment for those committed to a mental hospital, that "involuntary confinement without treatment [was] 'shocking' " and that a patient acquitted by reason of insanity and confined in St. Elizabeths Hospital was entitled to a hearing upon the allegation that he was denied adequate and humane medical care. The decision, however, provides no indication as to whether St. Elizabeths physicians will succeed in establishing the adequacy of their treatment facilities by testifying that what they administer is "environment" or "milieu" therapy, i.e. in lay language, that the privilege of breathing in the air of St. Elizabeths Hospital is treatment enough. Rouse v. Cameron, 373 F.2d 451 (D.C. Cir. 1966).

For a psychiatric reaction to the case, suggestive of this very possibility, *see* the news story in Washington Post and Herald, January 10, 1967 at B1 entitled "Holtzoff Fights Back in Insanity Case Appeal" which includes this paragraph: "Dale C. Cameron, superintendent of St. Elizabeths Hospital and Rouse's ward psychiatrist, Stray H. Economon, testified that Rouse's treatment is 'adequate, if not ideal.' They described Rouse as a sociopath who does not respond well to treatment and is aloof and uncooperative."

As long as a prison-like atmosphere exists at St. Elizabeths, and understaffing and overcrowding continue, the right to treatment proclaimed by the Court of Appeals in Rouse v. Cameron will remain illusory.

mental hospital by Gilbert and Levinson. They describe two types of staff orientation, *custodial* and *humanistic*:

> The model of the custodial orientation is the traditional prison and the "chronic" mental hospital which provide a highly controlled setting concerned mainly with the detention and safekeeping of its inmates. Patients are conceived of in stereotyped terms as categorically different from "normal" people, as totally irrational, insensitive to others, unpredictable and dangerous. Mental illness is attributed primarily to poor heredity, organic lesion, and the like. In consequence, the staff cannot expect to understand the patients, to engage in meaningful relationships with them, nor in most cases to do them much good. Custodialism is saturated with pessimism, impersonalness, and watchful mistrust. The custodial conception of the hospital is autocratic, involving as it does a rigid status hierarchy, a unilateral downward flow of power, and a minimizing of communication within and across status lines. . . .
>
> The humanistic orientations, on the other hand, conceive of the hospital as a therapeutic community rather than a custodial institution. They emphasize interpersonal and intrapsychic sources of mental illness, often to the neglect of possible hereditary and somatic sources. They view patients in more psychological and less moralistic terms. They are optimistic, sometimes to an unrealistic degree, about the possibilities of patient recovery in a maximally therapeutic environment. They attempt in varying degrees to democratize the hospital, to maximize the therapeutic functions of nonmedical personnel, to increase patient self-determination . . . and to open up communication wherever possible.[19]

Staff members of the John Howard Pavilion appeared characteristically deferential to standard symbols of authority. A leader of the bar representing an indigent client by appointment of the court could count on a greater show

---

[19] Gilbert & Levinson, *"Custodialism" and "Humanism" in Mental Hospital Structure and Staff Ideology*, M. GREENBLATT, D. LEVINSON AND R. WILLIAMS, THE PATIENT AND THE MENTAL HOSPITAL 22 (1957).

A similar phenomenon was noted in a southern state hospital. Ivan Belknap observed that "in its overall structure, the clinical system closely resembled a military command system, so closely, in fact, that a previous superintendent . . . used military terminology in communication with his staff, and punishment and privilege systems corresponding almost exactly to those of American infantry organizations." I. BELKNAP, HUMAN PROBLEMS OF A STATE MENTAL HOSPITAL 44 (1956).

of deference on the part of staff members than the recently admitted member of the bar performing an identical function.

Although nominal self-government for patients, including those of the maximum security John Howard Pavilion, has been secured, the respect relations between patients and physicians appeared far removed from those prevailing at the institution for criminal psychopaths near Copenhagen, where the medical staff joins the patients for their meals in the same dining room.[20]

Only minimal weight was accorded to the diagnostic opinions of junior psychiatric members at staff conferences preliminary to the certification of a given patient in a criminal case as with or without mental disorder, notwithstanding the fact that the senior physicians who seemed dominant spent half of their time in court and had clearly less contact with patients than the junior staff.[21]

It was commonplace for findings of psychopathology by St. Elizabeths psychologists to be rejected by the medical staff on the assumption that psychologists, like laboratory technicians, were only qualified to convey data, the true meaning of which could be detected only by the medical staff.

The matter is aptly exemplified by the testimony of a senior St. Elizabeths psychiatrist as to the insignificance of the opinions of all but the senior psychiatric staff members at such conferences in a recent trial:

---

[20] The Institution for Criminal Psychopaths at Herstedvester, under the supervision of Dr. George Sturup, was visited by the author. For one of numerous published descriptions of the Danish treatment of the psychopathic offender, *see* S. HURWITZ, CRIMINOLOGY 412-14 (1952).

[21] Junior staff members and psychologists at St. Elizabeths encountered by project staff members frequently manifested a humane concern for the patient as an individual and a sense of optimism about his therapeutic potential, much at variance from the attitude frequently conveyed by senior staff members.

THE DEFENSE: Doctor, who was at that medical staff conference?

THE WITNESS: Doctor Owens, myself, Doctor Dobbs, Doctor Crowley, Doctor Hamman, Doctor Mollett, Doctor Wise, Doctor Kerring, Doctor House, and a psychologist, Doctor Stammeyer.

THE DEFENSE: Did all of these persons express opinions as to the mental condition of the patient?

THE WITNESS: I believe they did. I don't know. Some of the names that I mentioned are residents in training and their diagnosis is made by invitation and of course does not carry any great weight. And not often they will defer offering any diagnosis. So I don't know exactly who offered a diagnosis and who didn't.

THE DEFENSE: When you say it was the majority opinion, you are speaking then of the senior psychiatrists on the staff.

THE WITNESS: That is correct.[22]

Ward visits by senior members of the staff had an aura of military inspections in which subordinate attendants reported on their charges and presented the appropriate front of cleanliness and decorum.[23]

Asked as to the presence of odors of human excrement on a ward in which an individual beneficiary of the insanity defense had been confined, a St. Elizabeths physician denied having ever personally detected such odors but declared that hospital procedures were such as to make it likely that the ward would "get itself cleaned up" preliminary to a visit by a senior staff member.[24]

---

[22] Transcript of Proceedings in United States v. Oscar M. Ray, Jr., Crim. No. 250-61, May 23, 1962, at 24-25.

[23] *See* I. BELKNAP, HUMAN PROBLEMS OF A STATE MENTAL HOSPITAL, at 65 (1956).

[24] Testimony of Dr. David W. Harris, Transcript of Proceedings, Tremblay v. Overholser, H. C. No. 288-61 (D. D. C.).

Psychiatric concepts of "dangerousness" appear significantly affected by the tactical uses to which testimony as to dangerousness can be put. When, for instance, Joan Tremblay, charged with public intoxication and committed to St. Elizabeths pursuant to an insanity defense foisted upon her by government action, sought release by *habeas corpus,* St. Elizabeths physicians testified that Joan Tremblay was sick and dangerous and that her "dangerousness" consisted of a proclivity to fall while under the influence of alcohol.[25] When Charles Rouse, charged with carrying a weapon without a license and found not guilty by reason of insanity (in much the same manner as Joan Tremblay) sought release by *habeas corpus,* St. Elizabeths physicians testified that he was sick and dangerous and that his dangerousness was manifested *inter alia* by sending several young women proposals of marriage while upon St. Elizabeths premises.[26] Dr. Economon of St. Elizabeths Hospital, testifying for the prosecution, proceeded to describe Charles Rouse in this manner:

> He is a person who has not been able to profit very much from past experience and present learning situations. He is a person who has no loyalties. He cannot get close to people. He cannot love. He pushes love and human warmth and fellowship away. He is an individual with a marked lack of a sense of responsibility to himself or to other people.
>
> Although intellectually quite superior, emotionally he is immature.
>
> He has made threats against my person, both directly when we are in private and indirectly behind my back when he's on the ward. He consistently and continuously harasses the staff, demeaning us, degrading us, and makes most unkind statements about all of us.
>
> It is this behavior of Mr. Rouse's which we must continually attempt to understand, yet reject, not rejecting the person himself. He persists in this even to this day.

[25] Tremblay v. Overholser, H. C. No. 288-61 (D.D.C.) Transcript of Proceedings, *passim.*
[26] Rouse v. Cameron, H. C. No. 287-65 (D.D.C. 1965) Transcript of Proceedings, Jan. 9, 1967, at 106-109.

. . . .

THE PROSECUTION: Dr. Economon, referring you, specifically, to your note in the hospital record on April 15, 1966,—
THE WITNESS: Yes.
THE PROSECUTION:—would you tell the Court about the incident which that note concerned?
THE WITNESS: Yes, I will. This concerns some letters of correspondence between Mr. Rouse and several young women who were, shall we say, pen pals, individuals whom Mr. Rouse has not met personally. A number of our patients do correspond with pen pals. Occasionally it gets out of hand.
Here we have an instance, or several instances in which the situation got out of hand most grossly.
Mr. Rouse had been writing letters and receiving them from pen pals. These letters are supposed to be between friends, friends by means of the written word, because that's all that you are able to accomplish at this point while hospitalized.
Mr. Rouse wrote letters which were full of lies, deceits and half-truths. I cautioned him about behavior like this and asked that he keep his correspondence limited to a pen pal basis. He did not heed this gentle admonition of mine, and it came to pass that on one day I received several letters from as many young women, stating that Rouse was interested in marrying them, that he was going to be released from the hospital, could they see him, could they help him, "here's a photograph of Mr. Rouse," "here are all of his letters," "Do you think that you should keep them, that I should keep them?"[27]

One cannot help but note that the diagnostic concept of illness emerging from a Rouse case stands in sharp and disturbing contrast with the diagnostic concept of illness which permits drug addicts, sex perverts and victims of

[27] *Ibid.*

delusionary and hallucinatory experiences to be consigned to the penal system on the strength of St. Elizabeths testimony. Much of this is documented at a later stage.

Preoccupation with Security

Regardless of staff intentions, the policies of a public hospital are affected to a greater or lesser degree by public pressures. It is obvious that a significant segment of the public expects the hospital to give security priority over treatment.

As expressed by an editorial comment:

> St. Elizabeths, of course, is essentially a hospital and a good one. But as the custodian of criminals who are committed under the Durham rule, it also serves in a very real sense as a prison.[28]

The escape of a "suspected rapist" from the premises of St. Elizabeths Hospital, to take that example, can be counted on to bring public demands for a tightening of security measures.[29]

Whether willingly or unwillingly, a public hospital under these circumstances tends to yield to such demands to a greater or lesser degree.

Dr. Szasz has put the matter aptly and succinctly in these words:

> Undoubtedly, many psychiatrists do not want to be jailers, and refuse to be. But it is clear that many enjoy that role. Others may want to be detectives, judges, or even executioners.[30]

The maximum security John Howard Pavilion has "steel bars and bullet proof glass."[31] The hypothesis that the

[28] Washington Evening Star, May 17, 1963, at A16.
[29] *See* Washington Evening Star, Oct. 3, 1963, at A-20.
[30] T. SZASZ, LAW, LIBERTY, AND PSYCHIATRY, 65 (1963).
[31] Washington Post and Herald, Oct. 24, 1963, at A-3.

"authoritarian personality" is more likely to be attracted to such an institutional framework on a permanent basis does not seem implausible.

Overt acknowledgment of the custodial role of the hospital has appeared at the highest level of formal authority within the hospital.

As expressed by Dr. Winfred Overholser, as Superintendent:

> The notion that a verdict of not guilty by reason of insanity means an easy way out is far from the truth. Indeed the odds favor such a person spending a longer period of confinement in the hospital than if the sentence was being served in jail.
> As a matter of fact, only about one in four who have been sent to the hospital under this rule have been released. Some may never be released.
> If the patient is treatable he will be treated: if he is not, society is thoroughly protected.[32]

As a matter of routine practice, St. Elizabeths Hospital requests the transfer of those it has certified as mentally ill to the District Jail pending the disposition of their charges. Patients who have been transferred at the request of the hospital administration have (within the experience of the Project) included certified schizophrenics and psychoneurotics. Thus, a senior physician at the John Howard Pavilion declared in an affidavit, furnished to the prosecution, that a patient suffering from "psychoneurosis, anxiety reaction with obsessive features" would not be harmed in the least by a few months imprisonment in the District Jail.[33] Attempts by defense lawyers to resist such transfers have generally met with failure in the face of the judicial assumption that the courts should not interfere with internal hospital administration.

---

[32] Statement by Dr. Overholser in AMERICAN WEEKLY, Washington Post and Herald, June 18, 1961, at 4.
[33] *See* Clerk's File, Sutherland v. United States, No. 16, 160 (D.C. Cir. 1961).

Rigid Ordering of Rank and Prestige Among Patients

Rank and prestige differences among members of the staff seem matched by rank and prestige differences among patients. Clearly the favorite group among patients is that against whom no criminal charges are pending.

It would thus be inconceivable for, say, the Dix Pavilion of St. Elizabeths Hospital, housing civil patients exclusively, to recommend the transfer of a schizophrenic into an overtly disciplinary and predominantly punitive environment, not geared to the therapeutic needs of such a patient, on the ground that he would not be harmed by such a measure. It is commonplace, however, for the John Howard Pavilion, largely housing patients under criminal charges, to recommend the transfer of a schizophrenic to the District Jail to await disposition of his charges if regarded as "competent to stand trial" by the staff psychiatrists upon the explicitly stated assumption that he would not be harmed by a few months imprisonment.[34]

Defense attorneys who have occasionally inquired about the transfer of clients from the maximum security pavilion to a less restricted ward have often been met with the argument that the *pendency* of criminal charges required greater caution in the administrative disposition of the patient than would be indicated otherwise.

There appears to be little reason, moreover, to question the conclusion of a former United States Attorney for the District of Columbia that the attitude of the senior psychiatrists at the John Howard Pavilion is one of skepticism whenever faced with a claim of mental disorder by a patient subject to criminal prosecution.[35] Perhaps it is this type of skepticism which is mirrored in the following colloquy be-

---

[34] *See* Hearings before Judge Walsh in United States v. Walter Johnson, Crim. No. 381-59, July 13, 1961.

[35] Acheson, *McDonald v. United States: The Durham Rule Redefined*, 51 GEO. L.J. 580, 588 (1963).

tween a senior staff member of the John Howard Pavilion and defense counsel in the course of cross-examination in the District Court:

THE DEFENSE: Doctor, I suppose in your experience you have had numerous—well, thousands of interviews and have you been at all times alert to the possibility that the subject was malingering?

THE WITNESS: In my particular work this is very much the case because practically all of the patients I deal with are those who are involved in some kind of criminal activity, so that I have to be aware of the fact that they may try to present a picture of themselves which would be self-serving. So, this is very much in my mind.

THE DEFENSE: And the very fact that they are involved in a serious criminal offense, like Stewart here, charged with murder, would form a very strong motive for him to malinger?

THE WITNESS: It might, yes, very definitely.

THE DEFENSE: Not merely you, but all psychiatrists are aware of that possibility, are they not?

THE WITNESS: Well, as I say, particularly in the work that we do. Those who see patients, for example, who come to the hospital voluntarily, are obviously less concerned with this problem than those who are sent to the hospital in connection with a criminal charge.[36]

In a word, all available data tended to reinforce the impression of the hospital and its administration as "custodial" in every sense of the word.

---

[36] Transcript of Proceedings, United States v. Willie Lee Stewart, *Crim.* No. 633-53 (D.D.C. 1962), at 2043-2044. Goffman observed that demeaning and discrediting statements about patients in general are a commonplace characteristic of descriptions of a patient's history and general appearance in the records kept at St. Elizabeths Hospital. *See* E. GOFFMAN, ASYLUMS 156-58 (1961).

This, then, was the context which gave life to decisions affecting the insanity defense in the District of Columbia. What emerged during the period of the project study was a national problem in microcosm.[37]

Diagnostic Procedures Dictated by Understaffing and Overcrowding

Commitments to St. Elizabeths for mental examination and observation are made routinely for a period of ninety days,[38] an extension of an earlier sixty-day period. As expressed by a District Court judge: "Unfortunately, mental examinations take at least ninety days under the present system. I do not know why they should take that long, but psychiatrists claim they need ninety days. . . ."[39]

St. Elizabeths has, since 1959, requested a minimal period of ninety days to afford its staff the time it deems essential

---

[37] There is no reason to believe that the St. Elizabeths scene is significantly different from that obtaining elsewhere. The impoverished public mental hospital has, in fact, been a national blight. *See* A. DEUTSCH, THE SHAME OF THE STATES (1948). *See also* materials cited regarding the inadequacy of the national mental hospital picture in Arens, *Due Process and the Rights of the Mentally Ill: The Strange Case of Frederick Lynch,* 13 CATHOLIC U. L. REV. 3 (1964).

[38] This applies to District Court cases only. Lower courts (dealing with misdemeanors exclusively at the time of the project) committed defendants to D.C. General Hospital, usually for a period of one month. In isolated instances there were District Court commitments to the D.C. General Hospital as well. Those acquitted by reason of insanity were invariably committed to St. Elizabeths Hospital under D.C. Code Ann. §24-301 (1955). Unlike the D.C. General Hospital, St. Elizabeths was thus both the examining—and, ultimately treatment or custodial center—for those claiming the benefits of the insanity defense. The interest of St. Elizabeths in preventing the intensification of already existing overcrowding of its facilities is therefore obvious. It is noteworthy, too, that the senior physicians in charge of court-ordered examinations at St. Elizabeths, unlike those of the D.C. General Hospital who performed the same function, were usually older men with apparently limited professional mobility.

[39] Official Transcript of Proceedings before Judge Holtzoff in United States v. Gilleo, *Crim.* No. 583-59, March 25, 1960, at 3.

for court-ordered mental examinations. In view of what is set forth below as to the scarcity of contact between St. Elizabeths physicians and their patients, it is problematic whether the ninety-day period of observation requested by the Hospital was motivated as much by a desire to enhance diagnostic intensity as by that of adding to the testimonial effectiveness of St. Elizabeths physicians.

St Elizabeths records do not reflect the precise number of times that a given patient has been seen by a member of the hospital staff.[40] Omissions in the records, one must note in this connection, reflect either a lack of contact with the patient or an attitude of skepticism leading, significantly, to underreporting.

In a project case in which the defendant had been certified by St. Elizabeths Hospital as without mental disorder, the defendant's mother informed counsel that the defendant had been subject to unusual forms of mistreatment by his father. She told of whippings, of threats to assault the boy with an axe and of punishment of the boy by sticking wires in his penis.

The medical staff conference concerning the patient, held on April 25, 1960, did not have the benefit of this information. The hospital record reported the defendant as describing auditory and visual hallucinations at the staff conference, with this comment as to the reaction of the staff: "The patient is not very convincing in discussing these alleged hallucinations nor are the members of the conference very much impressed with his belief of mental illness at certain definite periods of his life."

The information gleaned from the defendant's mother was communicated to the superintendent of the hospital after the staff conference. The hospital record thereafter showed that two weeks *after* the staff conference the social service branch of the John Howard Pavilion conducted an interview with the defendant's mother which provided the details

---

[40] Testimony of Dr. Owens, Rivers case described *infra*. Ch. VIII.

referred to above. Two days later, without any further review of the defendant's record at another staff conference, the defendant was turned over to the marshal for return to the District Jail—with an unaltered diagnosis of "no mental disorder."[41]

When appointed to represent John W. Jackson, Jr.,[42] upon a charge of murder at a somewhat late stage of the proceedings, counsel was confronted with the fact that St. Elizabeths had already certified the defendant as without mental disorder.

In an interview with counsel at the District Jail, the defendant seemed unable to engage in rational discussion of the charges. He repeated insistently that he wished to be tried, sentenced, and executed on the same day. The trial, which was subsequently "continued," was at that time scheduled to be held within a week, and the defendant asked whether he could be introduced to his executioner on that occasion.

Upon discussion of the case with a senior psychologist of the St. Elizabeths Hospital staff, counsel was informed that the psychological test results suggested a significant possibility that the defendant was a victim of organic brain damage. The history of the defendant included a recorded instance of a skull injury and some fugue-type states of purposeless activity. Since the defendant had not been subjected to examination by a neurologist and had not received the benefit of such specialized neurological procedures as an electroencephalogram, a pneumoencephalogram, or routine skull X-rays in the course of his examination at St. Elizabeths Hospital, counsel considered it essential to secure further information on that score. At that stage the defendant was subjected to psychological examination by a pri-

---

[41] A criminal case tried in the District of Columbia in 1961 and not identified in the interests of the defendant.

[42] United States v. John W. Jackson, Jr., *Crim.* No. 980-61 (D.D.C. 1962) at 445.

vately retained psychologist. An affirmative finding of organic brain damage was presented as the result of the new series of tests. Private psychiatric examination revealed a "borderline schizophrenic"—leaving the question of brain damage open. A private psychiatrist declared in an affidavit filed in the District Court that the defendant required "extensive neurological testing" which had not been carried out at St. Elizabeths Hospital.

When the St. Elizabeths staff was informed of these findings it responded in this manner as summarized in counsel's diary:

> At approximately 4 o'clock, on Thursday afternoon, May 17, 1962, I spoke by telephone with Dr. X of St. Elizabeths Hospital. I mentioned to him that several noninstitutional psychiatrists had reached a conclusion, differing from that of the St. Elizabeths Hospital staff, regarding John W. Jackson's mental condition. Dr. X told me that he was aware of this fact.
> He added that he did not see any point in having Mr. Jackson returned to St. Elizabeths Hospital, since he was satisfied that no different diagnosis would be made upon reexamination.

In one case, in which the defendant was charged with murder, mayhem, and rape, a motion for a mental examination was supported by affidavits. The affiants asserted, among other things, that the defendant had tried to kill himself with an axe, that he had laughed hysterically when alone, and that he had committed acts of bestiality with dogs.

When committed to St. Elizabeths for examination, the hospital authorities never contacted the affiants but certified that the defendant was "not suffering from mental disease at the present time" and that there was no "evidence of a mental disease" at the time of the alleged offenses.

The defendant did not attempt to interpose an insanity defense on the explicit assumption that his indigence made it impossible for him to challenge the institutional judgment of St. Elizabeths.

St. Elizabeths doctors told his court-appointed counsel that they had observed no behavior such as that described in the affidavits and that they could only report on what they observed on their premises.

The defendant was convicted of second-degree murder. The psychologist in charge of his case in the prison to which he was sent concluded that the sense of hopelessness generated by the sentence contributed to rendering the patient inaccessible to available psychotherapy.[43]

On occasion, however, a patient in the John Howard Pavilion receives observation and examination which approximates the ideal in the light of contemporary knowledge. For example, Bernard Goldfine, the financier, was seen by doctors at St. Elizabeths nearly every day, often for lengthy periods, after he had been adjudged incompetent to stand trial by the District Court of Massachusetts. The doctors also spent considerable time with members of the patient's family. The testimony of one of the examining physicians is eloquent as to what was done:

THE DEFENSE: Doctor, do you know the petitioner in this case, Bernard Goldfine?
THE WITNESS: Yes, I do.
THE DEFENSE: When was it that you first came to know him?
THE WITNESS: He was admitted to the hospital on October 18, 1960, and I saw him on that same day.
THE DEFENSE: Under what circumstances, if you know, was he admitted?
THE WITNESS: He had been admitted to St. Elizabeths as mentally incompetent to stand trial, as a transfer from the United States District Court of Massachusetts.

---

[43] The name of the case is deliberately withheld at the request of the prison psychologist who furnished the available information. The court files have been studied as well and are not identified for the same reason.

THE DEFENSE: Approximately how many times have you seen him, Dr. Owens, since the date of his admission to St. Elizabeths Hospital?

THE WITNESS: Well, it is hard to estimate the number of times because we don't keep an exact record of the number of times we see a patient. However, he is the type of individual, and with his illness, that he has, I have seen him almost, I would say, every day that I am at the hospital. I see him at least three or four times every week.

THE DEFENSE: Were there occasions when you saw him for as long as an hour?

THE WITNESS: This past weekend I saw him for one period of over two hours.

THE DEFENSE: On other occasions did you have protracted visits with him?

THE WITNESS: Yes.

THE DEFENSE: Approximately how many talks or discussions or conferences did you have with him that lasted for as long as half an hour?

THE WITNESS: Well, again, I would have to say, most of the time when you interview him it is almost impossible to complete an interview or discuss with him his difficulties in less than half an hour, so most of the interviews have been twenty to thirty minutes to an hour.

THE DEFENSE: Now, to your knowledge, were there other doctors attached to St. Elizabeths Hospital, and specifically to John Howard Pavilion, who interviewed him?

THE WITNESS: Yes.

THE DEFENSE: Who were they, sir?

THE WITNESS: The ones that I know of are, besides me, Dr. Platkin, Dr. Luik, and Dr. Read, and Dr. Dobbs, and Dr. Fogel. These are the ones attached to the John Howard Pavilion.[44]

---

[44] Transcript of Proceedings, In matter of Bernard Goldfine, Habeas Corpus No. 246-90 (D.D.C. 1960) at 36-37.

Another example is provided by the case of John Bradley, in which an unusual combination of circumstances, including the entry of private psychiatrists into the case, paid for by wealthy parents, resulted in a diagnostic study on the part of St. Elizabeths Hospital of far greater intensity than that which is carried out in the average case.[45]

Such cases tend to support findings by Hollingshead and Redlich that the kind of treatment administered to patients by psychiatrists depends to a significant degree upon the class and status of the patients under scrutiny.[46]

While this is in no way designed to suggest that class is critical in determining the quality of diagnostic studies done at St. Elizabeths, one is bound to record one's recollection of only a handful of cases of capital crime and/or insistent legal demands for diagnostic intensity as in any way approximating the quality of psychiatric study carried out for Bernard Golfine or John Bradley. Murder cases do in fact come to mind in which such intensity was absent.[47]

Operative Conceptions of Mental Illness

Consistent with its basic predispositions, the St. Elizabeths staff has rejected a significant number of personality and neurotic disorders as not rising to the dignity of mental illnesses.[48]

---

[45] A pseudonym has been used in *lieu* of the real name. The case is described in Chapter V.

[46] A. HOLLINGSHEAD & F. REDLICH, SOCIAL CLASS AND MENTAL ILLNESS *passim* (1958).

[47] *See* United States v. John W. Jackson, Jr., *Crim.* No. 980-61 (D.D.C. 1961). The Bradley case is discussed in a subsequent chapter.

[48] The "official" view of St. Elizabeths Hospital—propounded in terms of abstract theory and applied to the isolated case—has been in line with the AMERICAN PSYCHIATRIC ASSOCIATION'S DIAGNOSTIC AND STATISTICAL MANUAL. Thus, both "sociopathic" and "emotionally unstable" personalities have
(Footnote continued on next page.)

An examination of all criminal files in District Court throughout the calendar year 1961 indicates that St. Elizabeths certifications of mental illness rarely include non-psychotic disorders. It is fair to state that psychiatric literature points to a clear professional consensus as to the psychopathology of two types of offenders—often encountered in criminal practice—the chronic narcotics addict and the person persistently involved in the sexual molestation of a child.[49] This consensus, however, has not bound St. Elizabeths Hospital.

At a time when a presidential commission was urging understanding of narcotics addicts as medically handicapped, St. Elizabeths Hospital blithely certified a significant number of chronic narcotics addicts as without mental disorder. In so doing, St. Elizabeths physicians occasionally described such offenders as "mentally healthy."[50] In fiscal year 1962 nine narcotic addicts were pronounced free of any manner of mental disorder by St. Elizabeths. Another thir-

---

been officially proclaimed to conform to the hospital's conception of mental illness, in one case in mid-trial following a weekend conference by the hospital staff. *See e.g.,* In re Rosenfield, 157 F. Supp. 18 (D.D.C. 1957) *and* Campbell v. United States, 307 F. 2d 597 (D.C. Cir. 1962). The evidence however suggests the practical repudiation of this view in numerous court cases, particularly as the full implications of the acceptance by St. Elizabeths Hospital of all nonpsychotic sufferers of mental disorder hit home. It has been suggested—and it is borne out in terms of initial impressions that "what seemed to be emerging under the Durham rule was that neither legal principles nor medical concepts determined the defendant's fate so much as did administrative label changing by the hospital staff." Reid, *The Bell Tolls for Durham,* 6 J. OF OFFENDER THERAPY 58 (1962).

[49] *See* AMERICAN PSYCHIATRIC ASSOCIATION, DIAGNOSTIC AND STATISTICAL MANUAL (1952).

[50] *See* the testimony of Dr. David Owens in Rivers case discussed *infra* Ch. VII. *Cf.* White House Conference on Narcotic and Drug Abuse, Proceedings (1962); President's Advisory Commission on Narcotic and Drug Abuse, Final Report (1963).

For an example of a statutory scheme designed to substitute medical treatment for conventional punishment in the case of drug addicts, *see* New York Mental Hygiene Law §211-213 (1963).

teen of such addicts were diagnosed as suffering from mental disorders "not specifying use of drugs" and only two were diagnosed as suffering from a "mental disorder specifying use of drugs."

The following table as to the handling of narcotic addicts upon court-ordered mental examination by the John Howard Pavilion was furnished by the superintendent of St. Elizabeths to Professor Harold D. Lasswell of Yale University:

ADMISSION TO JOHN HOWARD PAVILION FOR EXAMINATION BY USE OF DRUGS AND PSYCHOLOGICAL DIAGNOSIS, FISCAL YEAR 1962

Psychological Diagnosis	Total	Not Addict	Addict Narcotic	Addict Other	Drug Use Unknown
Total	183	144	24	1	14
Mental Disorder specifying use of drugs	2	0	2	0	0
Mental disorder not specifying use of drugs	90	69	13	1	7
Without mental disorder	86	73	9	0	4
Diagnosis deferred or none given	5	2	0	0	3

In the same fiscal year, St. Elizabeths similarly certified a significant number of child molesters as without mental disorder. The following information was provided by the superintendent in reply to an inquiry as to the psychiatric diagnoses of child molesters upon the premises of St. Elizabeths Hospital:

1. There were 208 mental examinations given to prisoner patients admitted to Saint Elizabeths Hospital during fiscal year 1962.
2. Fifteen patients were charged with crimes involving sexual molestation and/or carnal knowledge of children.

3. Of these, six were diagnosed as *with mental disorder;* nine were diagnosed as *without mental disorder.*[51]

There appears to have been no significant change in the intervening years.

It is not facetious to observe under the circumstances that in addition to the mentally healthy chronic drug addict, St. Elizabeths appears to have discovered the mentally healthy sexual molester of children.

It would not be accurate to assume, however, that a victim of personality or neurotic disorder would never secure a certification as mentally ill by St. Elizabeths Hospital during the years of the project. Cases of such certification do exist.

It is impossible to provide meaningful criteria to enable an outsider to determine when a victim of a personality or neurotic disorder would secure St. Elizabeths certification as mentally ill. The availability of space coupled with the adjustment potential of the individual on a given ward may be significant factors. It would not be wise to assume that the wishes of the prosecution were irrelevant to diagnostic disposition. It may not be altogether accidental, therefore, that an individual diagnosed by St. Elizabeths as mentally ill by virtue of a sociopathic personality disorder[52] was viewed, on examination by a project psychiatrist, as "a quiet-spoken, friendly and charming" individual, whose adjustment potential in a prison or hospital environment appeared optimal.[53] Nonpsychotic conditions are more readily recognized as mental illnesses by St. Elizabeths when the consequence of such recognition is not an acquittal—but continued confine-

---

[51] Letter by St. Elizabeths staff member to Axel W. Oxholm, Esq. in Washington, D.C., dated October 9, 1963.

[52] *See e.g.,* United States v. Marocco, *Crim.* No. 208-62 (D.D.C. 1962).

[53] Report to Counsel, subsequently the basis of testimony by Dr. Leon Salzman, dated April 10, 1962, in United States v. Marocco, *supra.*

ment as, for example in the case of the hospital patient seeking release on *habeas corpus*.[54]

It is not altogether difficult to assess the philosophy underlying the rejection of most personality disorders by St. Elizabeths Hospital in the context of the insanity defense. Available evidence points to the probability that staff doctors balance the demands of pure medical judgment against the needs of hospital economics and administrative policy.

The matter has been aptly put in these terms by a senior staff member of the John Howard Pavilion:

> In clinical practice, private or institutional, the nosologic category of a patient is of secondary importance to the question of whether he needs help, whether he requires occasional, supportive therapy or intensive, investigative therapy. Not so with the psychiatrist in court, since he is there required to answer squarely and categorically whether, in his opinion, the defendant is or is not suffering from "mental disease." . . .[55]

It appears as though the senior members of the St. Elizabeths staff have assumed that this attitude enjoys the imprimatur of the Court of Appeals. This may explain why Dr. Julian, a staff psychiatrist at St. Elizabeths testified that a man may be mentally sick, but not sick enough to warrant a certification of a mental disorder for courtroom purposes.[56]

As expressed by a former United States attorney:

> there is reason to believe that the more experienced doctors [at St. Elizabeths] are reluctant to make a finding of mental disease without some evidence of its effect on conduct. They tend to look for behavior consequences, as one element of mental disease. . . .[57]

---

[54] *See* Tremblay v. Overholser, H.C. No. 288-61 (D.D.C.) Transcript of Proceedings, *passim* and Rouse v. Cameron, H.C. No. 287-65 (D.D.C. 1965) Transcript of Proceedings, January 9, 1967, *passim*.

[55] Platkin, *A Decade of Durham,* 32 MEDICAL ANNALS OF THE DISTRICT OF COLUMBIA, 317-319 (1963).

[56] Wilson case described in Ch. VI.

[57] Acheson, *McDonald v. United States: The Durham Rule Redefined,* 51 GEO. L.J. 580 (1963).

This table may shed light on some existing attitudes.

Psychiatric diagnoses of NGI admissions to Saint Elizabeths Hospital, by crime charged
[U.S. District Court, fiscal years 1954-1965]

Crime Charged	Total	Organic Disorder No.	%	Schizo-phrenic No.	%	Other Psychoses No.	%	Mental Deficiency No.	%	Psycho-neurotic No.	%	Personality Disorder No.	%	Without Mental Disorder No.	%
Murder	53	10	18.9	25	47.2	2	3.8	—	—	7	13.2	6	11.3	3	5.7
Rape	16	2	12.5	6	37.5	—	—	—	—	6	37.5	2	12.5	—	—
Other sex offenses	25	4	16.0	8	32.0	—	—	1	4.0	8	32.0	3	12.0	1	4.0
Manslaughter	6	1	16.7	2	33.3	—	—	2	33.3	—	—	1	16.7	—	—
Robbery	49	3	6.1	25	51.0	—	—	—	—	8	16.3	10	20.4	3	6.1
Aggravated assault	38	5	13.2	14	36.8	1	2.6	1	2.6	4	10.5	8	21.1	5	13.2
Housebreaking	49	2	4.1	23	46.9	1	2.0	—	—	9	18.4	13	26.5	1	2.0
Grand larceny	16	1	6.3	4	25.0	1	6.3	—	—	5	31.3	3	18.8	2	12.5
Forgery	31	2	6.5	6	19.4	—	—	—	—	7	22.6	15	48.4	1	3.2
Auto theft	28	3	10.7	12	42.9	—	—	1	3.6	5	17.9	4	14.3	3	10.7
Narcotics	30	2	6.7	8	26.7	—	—	—	—	3	10.0	16	53.3	1	3.3
Other felonies	20	2	10.0	8	40.0	—	—	1	5.0	3	15.0	6	30.0	—	—
Total	361	37	10.2	141	39.1	5	1.4	6	1.7	65	18.0	87	24.1	20	5.5

Source: Saint Elizabeths Hospital. [Abstracted from President's Commission on Crime in the District of Columbia, Report 541 (1966)—ed.]
Note: NGI stands for Not Guilty by Reason of Insanity.

An institutional psychiatrist, when asked to discuss a particular case in terms of mental illness and its causal relationship to crime, made this far-reaching admission:

> Sure, the man is sick. Under the *Carter* case, moreover, I would say that his crime is the product of mental illness. But I choose to accept a stricter legal standard because if I did not, we would be flooded with undesirables, who are not acutely ill and who would clutter up our facilities which are already strained to the breaking point.[58]

---

[58] Interview conducted by Project staff member with staff physician of St. Elizabeths Hospital, Aug. 21, 1960.

Yet another physician-administrator at St. Elizabeths Hospital stated in the course of an interview with a Project member that he was tending to be "conservative" in the evaluation of a patient to determine his mental state for courtroom purposes. There is much in the interview conducted in 1959 which explains operations at St. Elizabeths Hospital for that year, and indeed, far beyond that:

"He said he viewed the problem of causal relationship between crime and psychopathology as predominantly legal in character. Strictly speaking, he declared almost every action of some psychopathological character could be deemed the product of an individual's psychopathology. He gave the Dallas Williams case as an example. 'I, therefore, have to be much more restricted in my professional approach in the courtroom.' 'When the lawyers speak of product of mental disease or defect, I think of *M'Naghten*. There must be a direct, intimate relationship between crime and disease.' He thereupon proceeded to give several examples in which he believed an adequate causal relationship to have been established. Each involved a psychotic disorder including serious intellectual disorientation. He declared in this connection that where psychosis was involved the causal relationship between crime and psychopathology presented no problem."

Interview with Project staff member in 1959.

Still another characteristic series of responses was provided by a St. Elizabeths physician in 1959 in these terms:

"We are getting too many patients now. Putting them in St. Elizabeths Hospital might also be tantamount to a life sentence for a great many of them. Certainly this would be true of all the personality disorders. (These he considers untreatable.) This would be patently unfair in the case of the individual defendant acquitted of a minor crime like petit larceny by reason of insanity and characterized as suffering from a sociopathic personality disorder." While he regards the sociopath as devoid of mental disorder and characterized by only "willful quirks in his personality," a man who does not belong in a mental hospital, he goes on to say that if such a sociopath

(Footnote continued on next page.)

The statement of a private practitioner aptly portrays the situation in these terms:

> ... It appears to me that the government psychiatrists have been operating from the standpoint of *post-hoc* logic. That is to say—the determination of "mental illness" in a particular case is derived from two factors, (a) the available space, and (b) the treatability of the disorder recognized. I received the most significant part of my psychiatric training at St. Elizabeths Hospital, and can therefore see that side of the question. But it seems illogical for me that the fate of a man, standing accused, should be determined by logistic factors irrelevant to the life of this man...[59]

Contacts With the Prosecution and Suspicion of the Defense

Upon commencement of a court ordered mental examination, St. Elizabeths "routinely" requests background information on its patient from the office of the public prosecutor. Moreover, hospital records seem obtainable by members of the U.S. Attorney's office, whether by subpoena, court order or otherwise—well in advance of trial—often when the records do not appear available to the defense. In at least two instances defense counsel discovered hospital records of his clients in the possession of a member of the prosecution staff in advance of trial and was permitted to

---

is acquitted by reason of insanity, he, for one, would never authorize his release as cured.

Asked as to his view concerning a dynamic interpretation of crime, he replied that neither judge nor jury was competent to understand psychodynamics and that it was improper of the court to ask psychiatrists to talk only in dynamic terms. The jury clearly prefers clinical description. There has been, as far as he is concerned or aware, no basic change in the diagnostic practices at St. Elizabeths since *Durham*.

Interview with Project staff member in 1959.

[59] Letter to author, dated July 2, 1963. The identity of the psychiatrist who wrote it is kept confidential at his request.

inspect them only in the prosecutor's office. This experience does not seem to be unique.

Lawyers engaged in tort litigation obtain hospital records of their clients upon the basis of a written authorization by the clients as a matter of course. A written authorization by the client will, however, fail to secure the necessary hospital records from St. Elizabeths Hospital in a criminal case in the District of Columbia. Nothing short of a court order will succeed in obtaining the hospital records for the defense and the attempt to secure such an order may well be met by the hospital staff with opposition and dilatory tactics.

Attempts by defense counsel to secure supplementary information, beyond the conclusory statement of "with" or "without mental disorder" transmitted in the hospital official certifications, have met with differing degrees of cooperation and noncooperation by the hospital staff. While there have been occasions when explanatory statements concerning a given diagnosis were promptly and courteously provided, there have been other occasions when cooperation was utterly wanting on the part of senior members of the hospital staff. On one occasion, when defense counsel telephoned to inquire as to the specific diagnosis in the case of a defendant who had been certified as incompetent to stand trial, he was told by a senior physician of the John Howard Pavilion: "The District Attorney's office does not like us to engage in discussions of this kind with defense counsel."[60]

A lawyer who expresses his dissatisfaction with existing hospital procedures to a St. Elizabeths physician may be startled to discover that the prosecutor's office has been notified of his misconduct. A lawyer who had the temerity

---

[60] Telephone conversation between Project staff member and St. Elizabeths physician, Sept. 21, 1961.

to suggest, at the conclusion of a case, that the testimonial assertion that there are "mentally healthy drug addicts" was questionable and that the matter would be best verified by transmitting a transcript of such testimony to the American Psychiatric Association, was formally accused of "intimidation" on complaint of an outraged St. Elizabeths staff.[61]

Communication of Diagnosis

Preliminary to trial, St. Elizabeths communicates its findings in criminal cases in a form letter.

As late as 1960, the Hospital provided a modicum of background information on a patient within the form letter. When such explanations were provided, one would frequently encounter statements such as this:

> Although the patient is not well integrated, he does not show clinical evidence of overt psychosis or any other type of mental disease at the present. . . . Our findings and information are not sufficient to warrant the formation of an opinion that the patient was suffering from mental disease between February 29 and June 27, 1960. However, in view of the patient's personality organization and rather poor integration, the possibility of his being mentally ill during the specified period cannot be definitely excluded.[62]

Or this:

> Available information indicates that . . . [the patient] has been a poorly adjusted individual, showing schizoid tendencies, a poor marital adjustment, an unstable occupational adjustment, and a long-standing tendency to overindulgence in alcohol. However, in our opinion, he does not deviate sufficiently from normal to warrant a diagnosis of mental disease, nor do we find evidence of

---

[61] Rivers case discussed in Ch. VII.
[62] St. Elizabeths certification in United States v. Aloysius Hart, *Crim.* No. 661-60 (D.D.C. 1961).

mental disease existing on or about June 29, 1960. He is at best of dull normal intelligence, although he does not suffer from mental defect.[63]

At no time did the St. Elizabeths certification, however, provide the detail or the attempt at dynamic understanding of the individual exemplified by the certification of the D.C. General Hospital staff in the days when the latter still received cases from the District Court.[64] Significantly, during the last ten years, the form letter sent by St. Elizabeths has changed: no longer is any information given which might suggest doubts concerning the diagnosis of "with" or "without" mental disorder which is transmitted to the court. The letter is barren of all information except that contained in the conclusory statement. Although the certification may not reflect unanimous staff opinion, it never includes a reference to any dissenting view. Instead it conveys the impression of intensive studies, suggestive of numerous and detailed diagnostic contacts and private interviews.

A characteristic form letter from St. Elizabeths, communicating a finding of mental disease and its causal relationship with the crime in issue,[65] is brief:

> Mr. Morris Allen Kent, Jr. (Criminal Number 798-61), was committed to Saint Elizabeths Hospital on January 8, 1962, for a period not to exceed ninety days, upon an order signed by Judge Matthew F. McGuire, to be examined by the psychiatric staff of this hospital. It was further ordered that a written report be submitted to the court regarding the patient's mental condition; mental competency for trial; mental condition on or about June 5 and 12, and September 2, 1961; and causal connection between the mental disease or defect, if present, and the alleged criminal acts.
>
> Mr. Kent's case has been studied since the date of his admission to Saint Elizabeths Hospital and he has been examined by qualified

---

[63] United States v. Pee, Jr., *Crim.* No. 701-60 (D.D.C. 1961).
[64] A cutoff point around 1960 resulted in the routine referral of all mental examinations to St. Elizabeths Hospital.
[65] United States v. Kent, *Crim.* No. 798-61 (D.D.C. 1963).

psychiatrists of the medical staff of this hospital as to this mental condition. On April 4, 1962, Mr. Kent was examined and his case reviewed in detail at a medical staff conference. We conclude, as the result of our examinations and observation, that Mr. Kent is mentally competent to understand the nature of the proceedings against him and to consult properly with counsel in his own defense. It is our opinion that he is suffering from mental disease at the present time, Schizophrenic Reaction, Chronic Undifferentiated Type; that he was suffering from this mental disease on or about June 6 and 12, and September 2, 1961; and the criminal acts with which he is charged if committed by him, were the product of this disease. He is not suffering from mental deficiency. It is therefore requested that arrangements be made to have Mr. Kent transferred to the District of Columbia Jail to await disposition of the charges pending against him.

                              Cordially yours,
                              /s/ WINFRED OVERHOLSER, M.D.
                              Superintendent

How does this analysis compare with the certification made by the District of Columbia General Hospital psychiatric staff in the past and in those isolated instances in the present in which it is asked to pass upon a patient's mental condition for the District Court? D.C. General Hospital does not use a form letter. Frequently, a report by the D.C. General Hospital staff to the court does not provide a definitive opinion as to whether a given individual has suffered from a mental disease productive of a crime. In such letters there may be, however, a significant amount of background information susceptible to the development of an insanity defense. Such information most frequently highlights significant aspects of the patient's history. This in turn may be related to the current diagnostic view. What emerges may give rise to further defense contacts with D.C. General Hospital doctors and the possible assertion of an insanity defense on new grounds.

Perhaps the contrast between the D.C. General Hospital certification in District Court cases and that provided by St. Elizabeths Hospital at this time is best appreciated by juxtaposing the St. Elizabeths Hospital finding of mental illness in the *Kent* case, reproduced above, with that of the D.C. General Hospital in the same case. The letter of the D.C. General Hospital reads as follows:

> On October 17, 1961, Morris Kent, a sixteen year old, light skinned, negro boy was admitted to the District of Columbia General Hospital for mental observation. He was accused of taking part in a series of house-breaking and rape episodes. The question was raised as to the competency of this boy or the presence of mental illness that might have led to the crimes.
> Morris has been here for almost sixty days. During that time he has been seen by many psychiatrists, has taken part in a diagnostic study, including psychologicals, electroencephalogram, and projective tests involving art materials. In addition there has been constant supervision of his activities by nurses, attendants, and students all of whom are trained observers. There have been a series of staff conferences concerning all of the issues.
> It is the consensus of the staff that Morris is emotionally ill and severely so. In view of the many facets of his behavior we feel that he is incompetent to stand trial and to participate in a mature way in his own defense. His illness has interfered with his judgment and reasoning ability, and when faced with situations unfamiliar to him, his anxiety occasionally becomes so great he becomes disorganized. There are many examples of this including his inability to report blood on his penis, the fact that occasionally his clothes have been stained by a bowel movement and particularly the disorganized and almost incoherent way that he has presented the details of his life and the trouble he has had. In some ways he can appreciate the predicament he is in while in other ways his attitude contains disregard for what he has done.
> Indeed he has a mental illness of the schizophrenic type. At times this illness allows him to react within the bounds of normality, while at other times he reacts abnormally. During the time he committed the crimes his condition seemed to be a psychotic one but I am unable to arrive at a definite opinion on this matter. His life has been troubled for a number of years and has brought him great pain. Whether or not he can make use of psychotherapy is another issue, but it is our opinion long term treatment should be offered to him.
> We would particularly stress the idea that this is a dangerous boy. His behavior has become more pressured from within, and has included activities that can result in destruction to himself and/or others. Certainly close and constant supervision must be, it seems to us, the outcome of the interest in this boy. We would recommend that such placement take place in an institution allowing some treatment of his mental condition rather than incarcera-

tion in a jail. We cannot, however, ignore our responsibility in underlining the danger and potential damage to himself and others that lies within him.

Sincerely yours,

MARY V. MCINDOO, M.D. WILLIAM J. NOVAK, M.D.
Chief Psychiatrist Clinical Director in Psychiatry

In a word, the evidence suggests that the D.C. General Hospital certification tries to provide maximal information and does not bespeak a commitment to a guilty or not-guilty finding; the St. Elizabeths certification, in contrast, seems committed to a given end within the legal arena and is conclusory in the extreme in its formulation. Communication of a diagnosis is thus seen as a tactical weapon in its own right.

Awareness of the tactical uses of psychiatric information is most strongly highlighted in the psychiatric testimony of physicians from St. Elizabeths Hospital in open court.

Testimonial Practices

Most lawyers regard St. Elizabeths physicians as "good witnesses." These physicians gear their testimony to meet the psychological demands of the courtroom. In contrast to many private practitioners, they appear brief, succinct, and usually grammatical in courtroom testimony. Their testimony in fact often has the thrust of a good lawyer's argument on appeal. In this context, the striking fact is that St. Elizabeths physicians prefer to deliver their testimony in terms of the *M'Naghten* rules, often with marked facility.[66]

---

[66] This is known to any lawyer with significant experience in the conduct of the insanity defense in the District of Columbia. Prosecuting counsel frequently couch questions in terms of the "right-wrong" test and St. Elizabeths physicians have answered such questions without difficulty. The following is characteristic:

(Footnote continued on next page.)

The conception of partisanship, entertained by some of the St. Elizabeths staff, has been expressed by Dr. Mauris M. Platkin, a senior physician at the John Howard Pavilion of St. Elizabeths Hospital, in these words:

> Whatever the testimony of the psychiatrist, he will have previously determined in his own mind whether the defendant is suffering from a mental illness, and his testimony will inevitably be 'slanted' to lead the jury to the same conclusions as his own.[67]

A major characteristic of such testimony is its conclusory form. Explanation of a given condition and how it arose, developed, and affected the mental and emotional processes of the defendant is minimal. Supporting data are predigested for the jury and the final conclusion of "with" or "without mental disorder" is stated with maximum emphasis.

Unlike most of the private psychiatrists encountered in the courtroom, St. Elizabeths physicians depend overtly and overwhelmingly upon the hospital record of the patient for their testimony. The hospital record is perused repeatedly in the course of their testimony both on direct and cross-examination. As one listens to their testimony, one is clearly impressed with the legal virtuosity of the claim—usually of lack of mental disorder—which is propounded.

Q. Doctor, in your opinion was the defendant James Rivers able to distinguish right from wrong on December 15, 1961.

A. Yes.

Q. In your opinion, Doctor, could the defendant James Rivers embrace the right and resist the wrong?

A. In my opinion I would say that he could. This is what I believe to be a temporary situation with him, that he could postpone his immediate act, a temporary postponement because drug addicts in general, if on drugs, they have a craving, a tremendous urge to obtain the medication that they are receiving and I think they can postpone temporarily this desire but they eventually have a tremendous urge and a desire to satisfy the need, both physiological and psychological, to obtain the medication or narcotics.

PROSECUTION: Thank you, Doctor, no more questions.

Rivers case described in Ch. VII.

[67] PLATKIN, *A Decade of Durham,* 32 MEDICAL ANNALS OF THE DISTRICT OF COLUMBIA, 317-319 (1963).

The flesh and blood individual who is asserted to be with or without mental disorder rarely emerges from such testimonial utterances. The testimony is nonetheless presented with an air of certitude which has an obvious appeal to the lay mind.[68]

On most occasions, St. Elizabeths physicians will stress reliance upon what they describe as elaborate diagnostic studies but the quantitative character of diagnostic contacts will remain unstated except for those relatively rare occasions when opposing counsel will seek to exact specific answers on cross-examination.[69]

Although background information as to the defendant will often be sketchy, the testimony of the typical testifying doctors drawn from the John Howard Pavilion (the maximum-security wing of St. Elizabeths) will tend to dwell upon the various phases of a seemingly elaborate diagnostic work-up, even if the testifying witness has not participated in every such phase. It is not infrequent for such a witness to devote one-third of his testimony to describing his professional qualifications and the balance of his testimony, save for the conclusion of "with" or "without mental disorder," to describing each phase of the diagnostic work-up at St. Elizabeths Hospital—even to the mention of serology and X-rays.

The courtroom slant, as described by Dr. Platkin, is near hypnotic in impact. Hearing of X-ray studies in such a

---

[68] *See e.g.,* observation of C.J. Connolly & P. McKellar:
"When questions of testimony are involved, our legal informants have the strong impression that the court—that is to say the jury, judge, etc.—tend to be more impressed by the witness who can give his evidence with 'absolute certainty.' The witness who qualifies his statements and makes minor reservations for the sake of greater accuracy makes relatively less impact. This may not seem unreasonable but we know from many laboratory experiments that certainty is no absolute guarantee that the witness is correct or any more accurate."
C. J. Connolly & P. McKellar, *Forensic Psychology,* 16 BULLETIN of the British Psychological Society (No. 51, reprint) 3 (1963).

[69] *See* Rivers case discussed *infra* Ch. VII.

context, the average member of the courtroom audience thinks immediately of rationally relevant roentgenology—and assumes that skull x-rays have been taken. All too rarely does the bubble burst. When it does, impressive X-ray studies of the brain shrink to the standard chest X-ray of the routine "physical" on cross-examination.

The emerging legalistic virtuosity of St. Elizabeths psychiatrists' testimony is often coupled with unyielding and apparently irrational rigor. One example is provided by the Rivers case. Disclosure by defense counsel of a suicidal attempt by the defendant (conceded to be a narcotic addict) in no way deflected a senior St. Elizabeths psychiatrist from his opinion that the defendant suffered from no mental disorder, and was in fact an "emotionally healthy" person.[70]

Another example is provided by the *Ray* case. There, a senior physician of St. Elizabeths Hospital testified that epilepsy was a mental disorder only when it was clearly attributable to a "chronic brain syndrome," and that idiopathic epilepsy was therefore no mental disorder at all.[71] He did not know that the defendant had or claimed to have a history of delusions. When asked to assume such a history on cross-examination, he refused to admit that it could raise a reasonable doubt as to the accuracy of his diagnosis of no mental disorder:

THE DEFENSE: And you were unaware of the fact that . . . [an employer] describes him, his personality before he went to D.C. General Hospital, as one of the hardest workers she had, . . . that he got along well with everyone, and the guests, and then describes his personality after he returned from D.C. General Hospital, in March of 1960, in terms of, quote, "that the whole world was against him, and finally even me"; that God was telling

---

[70] The case is discussed in Chapter VII.

[71] United States v. Ray, *Crim.* No. 250-61, Official Transcript of Testimony of Dr. Platkin and Dr. Owens (D.D.C. 1962) p. 64.

him to do everything when he came back, and after she criticized him and told him to do something that he wasn't doing, he replied that God told me to do this; and on another occasion, when she reprimanded him, he replied that God and I are laughing at you; and that he often refused to go into the dining room because people were after him and some of the guests were Russian spies; and that he would giggle and laugh at nothing; and that because of this, and because of her opinion that he was mentally ill, she had to let him go, despite the fact that she was sympathetic and had done what she could to help him. You were unaware that she says that all of this took place after he was released from D.C. General Hospital for a period up to about the last of April of 1960; is that correct?

THE WITNESS: That is correct.

THE DEFENSE: Now this information, had it been in your possession, would have had to have been evaluated for its psychiatric significance, wouldn't it?

THE WITNESS: Yes, I would have evaluated it.

THE DEFENSE: And it has some psychiatric significance, right?

THE WITNESS: Any information concerning a patient is of psychiatric significance.

THE DEFENSE: Well, Doctor, let me ask you this: Assuming that this information were given you, assuming you believe that information, and assuming there was nothing to suggest that this behavior was the result of alcoholism or any toxic condition making that assumption, would you have an opinion as to whether or not the man was suffering from a mental disease at the time this behavior was taking place?

THE WITNESS: Would you repeat the question? I am not clear. Leaving out—

THE DEFENSE: I will be glad to repeat it.

THE COURT: The reporter can read it.

(The pending question was read by the reporter.)

THE WITNESS: What my opinion would be, that this is not in itself diagnostic of mental illness. I think some of the things you described were rather bizarre. But I think you have to consider, in obtaining information, how it is obtained, the way that it is related to you, by whom given; and other details that are going on within the patient at the time these symptoms were supposed to be present. So I don't think really on the information that you have given me, assuming that all of it is correct, that I would make a psychiatric opinion on the basis of the information that you gave me.[72]

Yet another example is provided by the fifth trial of Willie Lee Stewart on a charge of murder. Stewart had entered a grocery store at about closing time. After ordering a soda and a bag of potato chips which he ate in the store, he pointed a pistol at the proprietor who was standing behind the counter with his wife and daughter. The women pleaded with Stewart to "take the money" and offered him the register. He, however, "didn't step back, he didn't step forward, he didn't change expression, he just fired." Only then did he open the register "and emptied it very calmly, walked out the door and closed it behind him."[73]

Called as a government witness in that trial, Dr. Platkin testified that he had found the defendant without mental disorder. Upon cross-examination, he was informed by the defense counsel—clearly for the first time—that the defendant had engaged in various episodes of irrational violence, highlighted by an attempt at throwing his child into a blazing furnace. Part of the colloquy between defense counsel and Dr. Platkin went as follows:

THE DEFENSE: Suppose after that interview you had been told and believed that on two occasions in two different

[72] *Id.* at 43-45.
[73] Washington Post & Herald, March 14, 1953, at 11.

homes Stewart tried, actually tried, to put his little baby in a burning fire and was prevented only by physical intervention by at least one person, maybe two or three, and that on another occasion he gave every indication of wanting to throw his baby out the window and was again prevented only by physical force from doing so; suppose you believed he did those things, would you classify him as normal?

THE WITNESS: I would classify him as a person who has a vicious temper. I don't think on the basis of those two episodes only, and assuming—I had investigated those things, and I say this because whenever I receive a report like that, one of the things I am concerned about was: Was there alcohol involved; was he febrile, a person under a fever perhaps could behave somewhat irrationally; was there any other condition surrounding this event that might have caused him to behave this way. I don't think I could take it at face value and draw conclusions from that, but—

THE DEFENSE: Suppose—I'm sorry. Have you finished?

THE WITNESS: Yes; go ahead.

THE DEFENSE: Suppose you eliminate those possibilities? suppose he wasn't drunk, nor anything else of the sort you have mentioned. Do you still say that is the action of a normal man who is angry?

THE WITNESS: I'd say it's the action of a person with an ungovernable temper, but I wouldn't necessarily conclude at all that this is a mentally ill person.

THE DEFENSE: What do you mean, an ungovernable temper?

THE WITNESS: Well, a person who might want to throw his child out of the window or put him in an oven shows an extreme—extremely vicious temper which flares up, perhaps, based on some provocation, but it's not in itself evidence of mental illness.

THE DEFENSE: Do you mean ungovernable in the same sense that the word uncontrollable is used?

THE WITNESS: Uncontrollable with respect to the incident, yes.

THE DEFENSE: That's right.

THE WITNESS: Yes.

THE DEFENSE: A person who cannot control his temper is said to have an uncontrollable temper; correct?

THE WITNESS: Yes, that's correct.

THE DEFENSE: He does not have normal control over his emotions; is that correct?

THE WITNESS: Well, I don't know what you mean by normal, Mr. Murray. Very frankly, I know that many people, and again I include myself among them, at times display very irrational temperamental outbursts, some of which we are ashamed of afterwards, and yet at the time it's ungovernable we listen to no reason, we stop at nothing. The incident might last five, ten minutes, a half hour. And after that we recognize what we had done or tried to do, we recognize that it was not proper or acceptable or tolerable behavior. But I don't think it amounts to mental illness.

THE DEFENSE: You were referring, apparently, to a quarrel you might have with somebody in the house where you offend them by words. I am referring now to a man who tries to put his own baby in a burning furnace. Is there any difference?

THE WITNESS: Well, I wasn't referring to a mere quarrel. I was referring to something even more vicious than that. We get into fights. I don't include myself in this category. But we know many people who get into fights or have serious arguments in which physical violence is concerned, and it's regrettable, but we don't necessarily class these people as being mentally ill. As I say, it's a relatively frequent thing that people displace their hostility from other sources to areas where they will be less controllable. It's a common phenomenon that people come home and display severe outbursts of temper against relatively innocent members of the family after they have been chastened or scolded by the boss or have had an argument downtown or given a ticket by the policeman, or something like that.

I think it's asking too much to make a diagnosis of mental illness even when the outbursts of temper are of such degree of severity as you describe.[74]

To be sure, the Court of Appeals has at times indicated a healthy degree of skepticism concerning some of the "conclusory testimony" of St. Elizabeths physicians in some of the matters referred to above. Once the court declared that it had reservations about the validity of testimonial assertions by St. Elizabeths physicians that a "paranoid personality" disorder was not a mental disease.[75] But such times are few and far between.

Receptivity of Jurors and Judges to the St. Elizabeths View

What is the impact of such testimonial practices on such target groups as jurors and judges? Obviously, such practices tend to reinforce (perhaps critically) the preexisting attitudes[76] encountered among jurors and judges.

Further project studies illustrate that preexisting attitudes are indeed in tune with the orientation of St. Elizabeths.

Forty-nine jurors who had served in cases in which the insanity defense was propounded between 1960 and 1962 were interviewed after their release from jury duty. The selection of the forty-nine turned out to be haphazard insofar as a significant number of jurors refused to be inter-

---

[74] Transcript of Proceedings, United States v. Willie Lee Stewart, *Crim.* No. 633-53, at 2049-2051-A. (D.D.C. 1962).
[75] Rollerson v. United States, 343 F.2d 269, 272, n.6 (D.C. Cir. 1964). The court pointed out that the St. Elizabeths view appeared to be directly opposed to the views reflected in the DIAGNOSTIC AND STATISTICAL MANUAL of the AMERICAN PSYCHIATRIC ASSOCIATION and in standard psychiatric texts.
[76] *See e.g.*, R. J. SIMON, THE JURY AND THE DEFENSE OF INSANITY (1967).

viewed and the interviewing was cut short by intimations from the District Court bench that the practice was improper. As a consequence, the interviewing suffered from such disadvantages as the fact that some jurors were interviewed a few weeks and some almost a year after the conclusion of the trial, and that the sample was small.

The results gleaned from this inquiry must be stated with the reservation dictated by the limited numbers and resources described.

What was clear was that most (36 out of 49) jurors thought that mental illness was more likely to produce crimes of violence than crimes exemplified by the forgery of a check or the like. Only four jurors viewed a nonpsychotic mental disorder as capable of giving rise to a valid insanity defense. Characteristic quotations from such juror interviews were these:

> If he knew the difference between right and wrong, he would not have been insane.
>
> A check forger is a normal person in every way except he doesn't want to work for a living. He is not mentally ill.
>
> If his attack had been more immediate, I would have thought he was mentally ill.
>
> Drinking and homosexuality caused something in him to snap —at that instance he didn't know right from wrong, but I think he knew right from wrong soon after because he decided to cut his hair so that no one would recognize him.
>
> I don't think he was suffering from a mental disease or defect. I was convinced by the fact that, while being chased, he had the presence of mind to park the car, get out, and run into the house. If he was sick he wouldn't have run away.[77]

[77] A statistical analysis of the forty-nine jury interviews referred to above carried out at McGill University suggests that a negative correlation existed between the juror's attitude toward punishment and his understanding of the *Durham* rule. "The more punitively oriented a given juror was, the less he tended to . . . comprehend the *Durham* rule." Mr. Robert Reynolds, then a third-year student at the McGill Law Faculty, carried out this study with the use of a computer under the supervision of statistical specialists of the University.

It may not be irrelevant to note that a significant number of District of Columbia lawyers with substantial experience in the insanity defense
(Footnote continued on next page.)

Still under the auspices of the project, another attempt was made to probe the jurors' comprehension of judicial charges on the subject of the insanity defense. Student volunteers in sociology and psychology in three of the universities of the District of Columbia were read three charges deemed representative of the spectrum of judicial philosophy from pro to anti-insanity defense orientation and were then tested as to their comprehension of the subject matter. The range of accuracy was a little over one third.[78] The inaccuracies moreover were in line with the stereotype of madness of the eighteenth or nineteenth century.

The judicial audience was no less conspicuous for its failure to accord the insanity defense a sympathetic or understanding reception.

A content analysis was conducted of thirty jury charges in cases involving the insanity defense between 1960 and 1962 covering every judge on the District Court bench who had tried an insanity defense during that period. The analysis suggested that the judges, in varying but usually critical degree, had concentrated on cognition as the dominant criterion of exculpatory mental illness. The analysis demonstrated beyond serious doubt that the judges had explicitly maintained the verbal formula traditionally associated with nineteenth century interpretations of *M'Naghten*.[79]

Almost anecdotal usurpations of the psychiatric role by District Court judges in the cause of eighteenth or nineteenth century conceptions of mental functioning could be seen in open court.

---

have expressed the view that jurors would have little difficulty in accepting an insanity defense for a non-psychotic disorder if explicitly informed of their right to do so by the trial judge.

[78] *See Jurors, Jury Charges and Insanity*, 14 CATH.U. OF AM. L. REV. 1, (Jan. 1965).

The three jury charges utilized in the experiment are set forth in Appendix II.

[79] *See* Arens and Susman, *Judges, Jury Charges and Insanity*, 12 How. L. J. 1, (1966).

The following occurred in the *Jackson* case:

THE COURT: Do you know what day of the week it is?
THE DEFENDANT: The twenty-first, Your Honor.
THE COURT: Yes, the date. What month is it?
THE DEFENDANT: September.
THE COURT: What day of the week is it?
THE DEFENDANT: Friday.
THE COURT: Who is the President of the United States?
THE DEFENDANT: Mr. Kennedy.
THE COURT: Do you know who the Vice President is?
THE DEFENDANT: Lyndon Johnson.
THE COURT: And do you know where Washington is in the American League?
THE DEFENDANT: Yes, sir.
THE COURT: Where are they?
THE DEFENDANT: Last place.
THE COURT: He hasn't lost contact with reality. This motion says that he has lost contact with reality. I think he is in very close contact with reality. And that he has lost interest in the outside world which he has not shown here.
MR. ANDERSON (Counsel for defendant): He has also filed an affidavit that he was taking dope steadily during that period and he believes that has affected his mind.
THE COURT: He has read in the papers about California. No, I will deny the motion without prejudice. Thank you.[80]

The following in turn occurred in the *Washington* case, heard by the same judge, directly on the heels of *Jackson*:

MR. PITTS (Counsel for defendant): I haven't much more to add to the motion that is already in the record, Your Honor.

---

[80] United States v. James D. Jackson, Crim. Nos. 556-62 and 557-62, Proceedings before the Honorable Matthew F. McGuire, Chief Judge, on September 21, 1962 (D.D.C. 1962).

THE COURT: I will ask him the same question I asked the other man. Do you know what day of the week this is?
THE DEFENDANT: Friday.
THE COURT: Do you know the date and the month?
THE DEFENDANT: No.
THE COURT: Do you know who is President of the United States?
THE DEFENDANT: Kennedy.
THE COURT: Do you know who is the Vice President?
THE DEFENDANT: No. I don't.
THE COURT: Do you know where Washington stands in the American League?
THE DEFENDANT: I don't know.
THE COURT: I will refer this matter to the Psychiatric service of the Court.
MR. HANTMAN (Assistant United States Attorney): Very well.
THE COURT: If I sent him to Saint Elizabeths Hospital it would be three months before a report is made to the Court so I will refer this matter to the Psychiatric service attached to the Court.[81]

[81] United States v. Timothy Washington, Crim. No. 722-62, Proceedings before the Honorable Matthew F. McGuire, Chief Judge, on Sept. 21, 1962 (D.D.C. 1962).
Judicial hostility to the insanity defense is further expressed in such disproportionate questioning as a total of twelve questions addressed to five government experts and a total of 111 questions persistently expressive of incredulity in the good faith of the defense, addressed to defense experts in an insanity defense founded on drug addiction. In the case in which this occurred a defense psychiatrist was summoned—in full view of the jury—to the bench to answer questions concerning his fees and professional associations. He had been subjected before this to a battery of forty-seven questions by the trial judge.
See United States v. Horton, Crim. No. 59-62 (D.C. Cir. 1962).
In another case in which numerous psychiatrists were made available to an indigent youth of sixteen, charged with rape, a District Court judge declared with reference to some of the prospective expert witnesses for the defense that he "had a suspicion . . . that this [presumably the entry into the case of psychiatric experts outside the ranks of the public hospitals was] . . . a stimulated activity, and I am concerned about the activities of the
(Footnote continued on next page.)

Usurpation though this may be, one is bound to recall the marked deference with which St. Elizabeths testimony—and particularly such as is calculated to defeat the insanity defense—is received by the District Court. One is bound to recall also the nearly consistent judicial hostility, directed at legal as well as psychiatric champions of a liberalized insanity defense, further documented in the succeeding chapters. One is further bound to recall that the Court of Appeals has refused to interfere with convictions resting upon judicial charges freighted with cognition as the critical criterion of exculpatory mental illness—notwithstanding earlier lip service to quasi-psychoanalytic models in the handling of the criminal insanity defense.

The Quality of Justice Under Durham

Any survey of the scene makes it plain that the St. Elizabeths staff has engaged in no less than the usurpation of juroral and judicial roles by extra-diagnostic decision-making.

This has been observed by such distinguished critics of the *Durham* rule as Judge Irving R. Kaufman who declared that in the District of Columbia "psychiatrists when testifying that a defendant suffered from a 'mental disease or

---

National Institute of Health and the Washington School of Psychiatry . . . [and] if that . . . [was] so, somebody . . . [was] going to get in serious trouble." The judge thereupon directed defendant's counsel to "advise" the District Court "by the end of the week" about the activities of the suspect Washington School of Psychiatry which had furnished the defendant with some of his prospective expert witnesses.

Proceedings before Chief Judge McGuire, Feb. 19, 1963, at 26, United States v. Kent (D.D.C. 1963).

One such expert was referred to at that time by the prosecuting counsel, without reproof by the presiding District Court judge, "as *that* Goshen from West Virginia, *that* Dr. Goshen, I mean . . . hooked up with *that* Washington School of Psychiatry. . . ."

Id. at 27-29. (Emphasis supplied).

defect' in effect usurped the jury's functions." Judge Kaufman noted in this connection:

> This problem was strikingly illustrated in 1957, when a staff conference at Washington's St. Elizabeths Hospital reversed its previous determination and reclassified "psychopathic personality" as a "mental disease." Because this single hospital provides most of the psychiatric witnesses in the District of Columbia courts, juries were abruptly informed that certain defendants who had previously been considered responsible were now to be acquitted.[82]

A disturbing question must be raised as to the role of St. Elizabeths in the administration of the insanity defense under any rule of criminal responsibility. Does the chronic housing and staff shortage of the hospital, to say nothing of the custodial and authoritarian orientation demonstrated by its staff, disqualify the hospital as an impartial arbiter of the existence of mental disease or defect in criminal cases? The question has been asked by no less formidable a protagonist of government psychiatry than Dr. Winfred Overholser while Superintendent of St. Elizabeths Hospital. Dr. Overholser had been ordered to assist in the psychiatric determination of the presence or absence of sexual psychopathy, as defined by District Law. The findings of such psychopathy would have resulted in the indefinite confinement of the individual patient at St. Elizabeths. Writing to the District Court about his misgivings as to the demand upon the time of his staff members in the execution of such a study and the possible conflict of interests arising under such circumstances, Dr. Overholser declared:

> The order directs me to appoint two qualified psychiatrists to examine him, presumably at a place and time of their choosing. I shall arrange to have this done, but there are one or two points to which I wish to invite your attention. Obviously, I have no right to appoint anyone who is not on the staff of the Hospital. Our doctors are all extremely busy taking care of the patients who are already here and I shall somewhat reluctantly comply with your instructions.

[82] United States v. Freeman, 357 F.2d 606, 621-622 (2d Cir. 1966).

Another point of propriety is one that I should like to raise, namely, whether it is proper that physicians on the staff of St. Elizabeths Hospital should be called upon to determine whether a person not now in the Hospital as a patient should be examined by them to determine whether he should be sent to the Hospital. In civil cases I am sure that a question of this sort would be raised and I wonder whether it is entirely proper, whether legal or not, to make such an arrangement in a criminal case. The points which are raised are perhaps moot. Nevertheless, I should be remiss if I did not invite your attention to them in the hope that this apparent conflict of interest may not arise again.[83]

An equally disturbing question which must be raised is whether the available pool of psychiatric "talent" in the District of Columbia is in fact sufficiently skilled and appropriately committed to the ideology of a democratic social order to permit constructive legal-psychiatric teamwork on any level in the reasonably foreseeable future.[84]

A survey of the scene is thought-provoking; it is not conducive to a sense of optimism or civic pride.

---

[83] United States v. Harry J. Allen, Crim. No. 438-60 (D.D.C. 1961).

[84] Whatever misgivings may arise on this score *vis-à-vis* government psychiatrists are fully matched by similar misgivings *vis-à-vis* significant numbers of private psychiatrists engaged in legal-psychiatric work in the District of Columbia. The interviewing of private psychiatrists in the nation's capital to determine their attitudes toward the insanity defense conducted by project staff members between 1959 and 1960 revealed a startling frequency in "custodial" and "punitive" orientation. Observation of such psychiatrists in court-work further revealed an equally startling appearance of indifference to the fate of the defendant and a disconcerting carelessness in the organization and presentation of testimonial materials. The bills submitted by some private psychiatrists erred occasionally on the side of self-interest. There were, of course, conspicuous exceptions.

Chapter IV

DUE PROCESS AND THE RIGHTS OF THE MENTALLY ILL: THE STRANGE CASE OF FREDERICK LYNCH

The insanity defense is a shield, most often wielded on behalf of the poor man charged with crime. It can, however, be forged into the sword of the prosecution and become an instrument of oppression on the part of the government. Frederick Lynch paid for such a defense with his life. Recounting his doomed fight for life, one is uneasily reminded of the warning uttered in 1928 by Justice Brandeis in dissent:

> Experience would teach us to be most on our guard to protect liberty when the Government's purposes are beneficent. Men born to freedom are naturally alert to repel invasion of their liberty by evil-minded rulers. The greatest dangers to liberty lurk in insidious encroachment by men of zeal, well-meaning but without understanding.[1]

Prior to his first and final encounter with criminal justice, Frederick Lynch, a respectable realtor and onetime lieutenant colonel who had served with distinction in the Air Force, lived in one of Washington's more exclusive and fashionable neighborhoods.

On November 6, 1959, Frederick Lynch was arrested and charged in the then Municipal Court for the District of

---

[1] Olmstead v. United States 277 U.S. 438, 479 (1928).

Columbia with a violation of the "Bad Check" Law.[2] Specifically, Frederick Lynch was charged with overdrawing his checking account by $100 with an intent to defraud, that intent being deemed inferrable by local law from his failure to make restitution within a period of five days after notice of the overdraft.

On November 29, 1959, Frederick Lynch, who, after a mental examination upon court order pursuant to D.C. Code Ann. § 24-301 (a),[3] had been pronounced mentally ill as of

---

[2] The Bad Check Law, D.C. CODE ANN. §22-1410 (1961) read as follows:

"Any person within the District of Columbia who, with intent to defraud, shall make . . . any check, draft, or order for the payment of money upon any bank or other depository, knowing at the time of such making . . . that the maker or drawer has not sufficient funds in or credit with such bank . . . shall be guilty of a misdemeanor and punishable by imprisonment for not more than one year, or be fined not more that $1,000, or both. . . . [The] making . . . by such maker or drawer of a check, draft, or order, payment of which is refused by the drawee because of insufficient funds of the maker or drawer to its possession or control, shall be prima facie evidence of the intent to defraud and of knowledge of insufficient funds in or credit with such bank or other depository, provided such maker or drawer shall not have paid the holder thereof the amount due thereon, together with the amount of protest fees, if any, within five days after receiving notice in person, or writing, that such draft or order has not been paid."

[3] D.C. CODE ANN. §24-301(a) (1961) read as follows:

"Whenever a person is arrested, indicted, charged by information, or is charged in the juvenile court of the District of Columbia, for or with an offense and prior to the imposition of sentence or prior to the expiration of any period of probation, it shall appear to the court from the court's own observations, or from prima facie evidence submitted to the court, that the accused is of unsound mind or is mentally incompetent so as to be unable to understand the proceedings against him or properly to assist in his own defense, the court may order the accused committed to the District of Columbia General Hospital or other mental hospital designated by the court, for such reasonable period as the court may determine for examination and observation and for care and treatment if such is necessary by the psychiatric staff of said hospital. If, after such examination and observation, the superintendent of the hospital, in the case of a mental hospital, or the chief psychiatrist of the District of Columbia General Hospital, in the case of District of Columbia General Hospital, shall report that in his opinion, the accused is of unsound mind or mentally incompetent,

(Footnote continued on next page.)

the time of the alleged offense but nonetheless competent to stand trial, sought to enter a guilty plea to the information against him. The presiding judge refused to accept the guilty plea and, acting over the objection of Frederick Lynch, duly represented by counsel, heard evidence upon the charges.[4]

In a trial in which the conventional positions of the participants were reversed, the defense sought to secure the "conviction" of Frederick Lynch, while the prosecution sought to secure his "acquittal"—significantly, by reason of insanity. Over the objection of Frederick Lynch, a government psychiatrist, called at the behest of either the court or prosecution,[5] testified that Frederick Lynch had been a victim of mental illness as of the time of the overdrawn checking account and that his crime, if any, was the product of his illness.[6]

---

such report shall be sufficient to authorize the court to commit by order the accused to a hospital for the mentally ill unless the accused or the government objects, in which event, the court, after hearing without a jury, shall make a judicial determination of the competency of the accused to stand trial. If the court shall find the accused to be then of unsound mind or mentally incompetent to stand trial, the court shall order the accused confined to a hospital for the mentally ill."

[4] Transcript of Record in the Supreme Court of the United States, at 25-26, Lynch v. Overholser, 369 U.S. 705 (1962).

[5] The lack of a transcript in the Municipal Court proceedings precludes determination as to whether it was the court or the prosecution which called the psychiatrist in the case.

[6] Since no transcript of the proceedings in Municipal Court was available, it is fair to assume that the testimony of the government psychiatrist was substantially the equivalent of the letter which he furnished to the court.

That letter read as follows:

"Dear Sir:

This patient was admitted to the District of Columbia General Hospital on November 6, 1959. On December 4, 1959 he was reported to the court as being of unsound mind, and unable to understand the charges against him.

Since the time of our report, Mr. Lynch has shown some improvement and at this time appears able to understand the charges against him, and to assist counsel in his own defense. In my opinion he was suffering from

(Footnote continued on next page.)

As a result of recent reverses, Frederick Lynch lacked the resources to secure independent psychiatric assessment of the claims propounded by the one psychiatrist concerning his "mental health." Accordingly, the judicial inquiry into Frederick Lynch's state of mind remained one-sided.

Frederick Lynch was thereupon—still over his objection—acquitted by reason of insanity.[7] Then and there the court, without holding any hearing or making any determination as to Frederick Lynch's then existing state of mind or need for hospitalization, ordered his commitment to a mental institution in accordance with D.C. Code Ann. § 24-301 (d) (1961)[8] until such time as he, pursuant to that law,[9] as then

---

a mental disease, i.e., a manic depressive psychosis, at the time of the crime charged. Such an illness would particularly affect his judgment in regard to financial matters, so that the crime charged would be a product of his mental disease.

At the present time Mr. Lynch appears to be in an early stage of recovery from manic depressive psychosis. It is thus possible that he may have further lapses of judgment in the near future. It would be advisable for him to have a period of further treatment in a psychiatric hospital.
Sincerely yours,
James A. Ryan, M.D.
Assistant Chief Psychiatrist."

Transcript of Record, *supra*, note 4, at 24.

[7] Transcript of Record, *supra*, 21, 25.

[8] D.C. CODE ANN. §24-301 (*d*) (1961) reads as follows:

"(d) If any person tried upon an indictment or information for an offense, or tried in the juvenile court of the District of Columbia for an offense, is acquitted solely on the ground that he was insane at the time of its commission, the court shall order such person to be confined in a hospital for the mentally ill."

[9] D.C. CODE ANN. §24-301 (*e*) (1961) read as follows:

"(e) Where any person has been confined in a hospital for the mentally ill pursuant to subsection (d) of this section, and the superintendent of such hospital certifies (1) that such person has recovered his sanity, (2) that, in the opinion of the superintendent, such person will not in the reasonable future be dangerous to himself or others, and (3) in the opinion of the superintendent, the person is entitled to his unconditional release from the hospital, and such certificate is filed with the clerk of the court in which the person was tried, and a copy thereof served on the United States Attorney or the Corporation Counsel of the District of Columbia, whichever office prosecuted the accused, such certificate shall be sufficient to authorize

(Footnote continued on next page.)

interpreted by the Court of Appeals, was deemed judicially and psychiatrically recovered from his illness and no longer prone (in the reasonably foreseeable future) to overdrawing his checking account.[10] Inevitably, the Municipal Court bypassed the procedural safeguards available to the citizen whose commitment is sought under the Civil Commitment Law.[11]

---

the court to order the unconditional release of the person so confined from further hospitalization at the expiration of fifteen days from the time said certificate was filed and served as above; but the court in its discretion may, or upon objection of the United States or the District of Columbia shall, after due notice, hold a hearing at which evidence as to the mental condition of the person so confined may be submitted, including the testimony of one or more psychiatrists from said hospital. The court shall weigh the evidence and, if the court finds that such person has recovered his sanity and will not in the reasonable future be dangerous to himself or others, the court shall order such person unconditionally released from further confinement in said hospital. If the court does not so find, the court shall order such person returned to said hospital. Where, in the judgment of the superintendent of such hospital, a person confined under subsection (d) above is not in such condition as to warrant his unconditional release, but is in a condition to be conditionally released under supervision, and such certificate is filed and served as above provided, such certificate shall be sufficient to authorize the court to order the release of such person under such conditions as the court shall see fit at the expiration of fifteen days from the time such certificate is filed and served pursuant to this section: *Provided,* That the provisions as to hearing prior to unconditional release shall also apply to conditional release, and, if, after a hearing and weighing the evidence, the court shall find that the condition of such person warrants his conditional release, the court shall order his release under such conditions as the court shall see fit, or, if the court does not so find, the court shall order such person returned to such hospital."

[10] *See* Overholser v. Russell, 283 F.2d 195 (D.C. Cir. 1960) for the Court of Appeal interpretation of §24-301 (e). For the action of the Municipal Court in this context *see* Transcript of Record, *supra* note 4, at 21, 25.

[11] The procedure for civil commitment in the District of Columbia was a relatively exacting one at the time of this case. It was set forth in D.C. CODE ANN. §21-306-14 (1961).

The forcible hospitalization of a mental patient was initiated by a verified petition alleging insanity filed by "any person with whom . . . [the] alleged insane person may reside, or at whose house he may be, or [by] the father or mother, husband or wife, brother or sister, or the child of lawful age of any such person, or the nearest relative or friend available, or the committee of such person, or [by] an officer of any charitable in-
(Footnote continued on next page.)

One is bound to observe at this point that there was no reason to believe that in overdrawing his checking account, Frederick Lynch had had any intent whatever to defraud anyone. How explain then his consistent and persistent attempt to enter a guilty plea to the charge of passing the bad checks?

The short answer is probably that his counsel, apprehensive of the weight of the statutory presumption of intent to defraud in any trial which might be held and hopeful of a suspended sentence on a minor first "offense," advised his client to elect a guilty plea to avoid the danger of a sentence on a finding of guilty or commitment on an acquittal by reason of insanity after the assertion of the insanity defense by the court or prosecution. The soundness of this view was in fact demonstrated by the very trial of Frederick Lynch.

Under established District of Columbia law, an acquittal by reason of insanity is conditioned upon the initial estab-

---

stitution, home, or hospital in which such person may be, or any duly accredited officer or agent of the Board of Public Welfare or any officer authorized to make arrests in the District of Columbia who has arrested any alleged insane person found in any public place." D.C. CODE ANN. §21-310 (1961).

The verified petition had to be "accompanied by the affidavits of two or more responsible residents [who have known the person whose commitment is sought], setting forth that they believe . . . [such] person . . . to be insane or of an unsound mind, . . . that they believe such person to be incapable of managing his own affairs, and that such person is not fit to be at large or go unrestrained, and that if such person be permitted to remain at liberty, the rights of persons and property will be jeopardized or the preservation of public peace imperiled or the commision of crime rendered probable, and that such person is a fit subject for treatment by reason of his . . . mental condition . . ." D. C. CODE ANN. §21-311 (1966).

The allegedly insane person was then entitled to an examination and hearing of his case by the Mental Health Commision. *Ibid.*

A report by the Mental Health Commission holding the patient to be insane called for a District Court hearing on the matter with a jury trial—if demanded by the patient. D.C. CODE ANN. §21-311, 312, 313, 314 (1961). The recently amended statute known as the Hospitalization of the Mentally Ill Act of 1964 has simplified these procedures without sacrificing essential safeguards. *See* D.C. CODE §21-501 *et seq.* (1967).

lishment of the substantive crime charged.[12] Frederick Lynch's "acquittal," was based initially upon the finding that he had been guilty of passing bad checks with intent to defraud. The intent to defraud under the circumstances seems to have been inferred from the failure of Frederick Lynch to make restitution within a period of five days after notice that the checks had been dishonored.[13]

Frederick Lynch's proffer of a guilty plea may be reasonably interpreted as the product of a careful estimate of the existing situation under the inevitably swift procedures which have characterized so many of our congested and understaffed courts of inferior jurisdiction.[14] Certainly, the rational as well as humane resolution of the dilemma posed by Frederick Lynch would have been the dismissal of the charges coupled with arrangements for appropriate medical care which might or might not, in the light of available family resources, have included the initiation of civil

---

[12] "Inherent in a verdict of not guilty by reason of insanity are two important elements, (a) that the defendant did in fact commit the act charged, (b) that there exists some rational basis for belief that the defendant suffered from a mental disease or defect of which the criminal act is a product." Ragsdale v. Overholser, 281 F.2d 943, 949 (D.C. Cir. 1960).

"The general verdict of not guilty by reason of insanity . . . [carries] with it a finding, except for the question as to his sanity [that] defendant was guilty as charged." Rucker v. United States, 280 F.2d 623, 625 (D.C. Cir. 1960). This finding may be based either upon independent evidence or stipulation. Psychiatrists, testifying that a "crime" was a product of "mental disease or defect" are not required to have established the existence of such a "crime" on their own.

[13] *See prima facie* evidence, provision, contained in Bad Check Law as reproduced in note 2.

[14] The impression thus gleaned is confirmed by the results of recent research.

"In the densely populated case-load of the metropolitan court, there is a special danger that some of the cases will be completed too fast, so that perfunctory, routine disposition will be made of some problems that should receive more prolonged or more specialized attention in order to achieve a just disposition." Virtue, *The Two Faces of Janus: Delay in Metropolitan Trial Courts,* 328 ANNALS 126 (1960).

commitment proceedings.[15] This was not to be. Frederick Lynch was proceeded against as an accused criminal and subjected to the summary commitment process of the criminal court.

On his arrival at St. Elizabeths Hospital, home to the beneficiary of the successful insanity defense in the District of Columbia, Frederick Lynch who had been taken from the care of a private physician (not a psychiatrist) by the long arm of fate, was housed with 1,000 other mental patients in a ward which provided precisely two psychiatrists for their "care and treatment."[16]

Acting at the behest of the American Civil Liberties Union, I sought to interview Frederick Lynch at St. Elizabeths Hospital, preliminary to the filing of a *habeas corpus* petition in his behalf in the District Court. I was informed at that time that the "patient" was working on a vegetable patch in an outlying area of the hospital grounds and that he would be unavailable for several hours, irrespective of his legal needs.[17]

A *habeas corpus* petition attacking his commitment, was finally filed on June 13, 1960. It asserted that commitment of Frederick Lynch pursuant to an involuntary insanity defense as outlined above violated due process of law. It fur-

---

[15] It is interesting to note that the concern of the prosecution for the maintenance of the unblemished civic record of the defendant did not become manifest at the commencement of the proceedings when the entry of a plea of *nolle prosequi* by the prosecution could have accomplished precisely that result.

[16] Lynch v. Overholser, Habeas Corpus 171-60 (D.D.C. 1960).

[17] The episode appears characteristic of the hospital *milieu,* described in a comparable context, in these words:

"In the mental hospital, the setting and the house rules press home to the patient that he is, after all, a mental case who has suffered some kind of social collapse on the outside, having failed in some overall way, and that here he is of little social weight, being hardly capable of acting like a full-fledged person at all. These humiliations are likely to be most keenly felt by middle-class patients, since their previous condition of life little immunizes them against such affronts, but all patients feel some downgrading." E. GOFFMAN, ASYLUMS 151-2 (1961).

ther asserted that the commitment of Frederick Lynch circumvented the safeguards of the Civil Commitment Law.[18] In the words of the *habeas corpus* petition:

> If this commitment be permitted to stand, the mere establishment of a reasonable doubt of mental health could result in the instant confinement in a mental hospital, without benefit of Mental Health Commission or District Court proceeding, including jury trial, of any citizen facing the Municipal Court upon the basis of a parking ticket. The Court of Appeals has expressed itself in unambiguous terms upon this issue in Williams v. Overholser, 259 F. 2d 175 (D.C. Cir. 1958).

After a hearing upon the writ, held on June 16, 1960, the District Court held that an improper circumvention of the Civil Commitment Law had taken place in the Municipal Court. In the words of the District Court Judge:

> I don't believe that the Municipal Court had a right to convert . . . the proceeding into a civil commitment proceeding, which is what it did. Therefore, I don't think the Municipal Court had jurisdiction to commit . . . [Frederick Lynch] to St. Elizabeths.[19]

In an order signed on June 27, 1960, the District Court sustained the writ and declared that:

> The Municipal Court lacked jurisdiction to effect such a commitment of the petitioner as of unsound mind by use of a criminal proceeding in substitution for civil commitment procedures established by law . . . [and] . . . that petitioner, therefore, . . . [was] illegally detained at St. Elizabeths Hospital.[20]

The District Court order, directing the release of Frederick Lynch, however, was stayed pending an appeal therefrom by the prosecution.[21] As required by the rules of the Court of Appeals, the prosecution filed a brief attacking the District Court's order directing the release of Colonel

[18] Transcript of Record, *supra,* note 4, at 3-5.
[19] *Id.,* at 18.
[20] *Id.,* at 20.
[21] *Ibid.*

Lynch as erroneous. In so doing it claimed that the Municipal Court exercised an unquestionable discretion in rejecting a guilty plea and went on to assert that a duty was in fact incumbent on the Municipal Court to reject the guilty plea in the light of such information of mental disorder as was made available to it. It declared that the fact that Frederick Lynch might be kept confined within St. Elizabeths Hospital for a period longer "than the maximum imprisonment possible under the offenses to which he desired to plead guilty," was not relevant to a determination of the legality of his detention. The brief then proceeded to assert that the purpose of hospitalization was both to provide Lynch with facilities for treatment and rehabilitation as well as to protect him and the public at large and went on to argue:

> Neither the ends of justice demanded by society nor appellee's rights as an individual citizen would have been properly served had he been tried on the charges and no effort made to disclose his mental condition when the acts were committed.[22]

Addressing itself to Frederick Lynch, it concluded:

> Therefore, accepting for the sake of argument the appellee's allegation of "a stigma of insanity," acceptance of his guilty pleas would have created a double stigma—conviction of crime and insanity.
> In sum, the way of justice is clear. There can be no normal justification for a judge of any court permitting an accused to plead guilty to a crime when the judge had excellent reasons to believe the accused did not have the mental capacity to commit the offense. To hold otherwise would be to violate one of the basic tenets of criminal law, and would have the courts and the Government standing idly by while a man went to prison who was mentally ill when he committed the acts charged and who was in need of hospitalization. True, he was competent to be tried. But he was still suffering from mental illness despite his competency to stand trial. This Court has unequivocally held that the standard of measurement of competency to stand trial is dif-

---

[22]Overholser v. Lynch, No. 15859, U.S. Court of Appeals for the District of Columbia Circuit, Brief for Appellant, at 20.

ferent from the standard of measurement for responsibility for a criminal act." . . . Therefore, it appears that if the Municipal Court was wrong in the instant case, it would not matter what criteria or tests were used to measure criminal responsibility when the accused is competent to stand trial and wants to plead guilty. It could be the *Durham* rule, the "right and wrong" standard, and indeed, even the "wild beast test"; so long as the accused standing before the court was mentally competent to be tried, he could plead guilty and go to prison. This result does not square with the public policy of treating such persons as appellee, who are seriously disturbed mentally and are in present need of treatment for their own good as for the good of society.

It necessarily follows that the Municipal Court was correct in refusing appellee's pleas of guilty and in hearing the testimony —including that of the psychiatrist. The Court did not lose its jurisdiction nor abuse its discretion at any time in the proceedings. In finding appellee not guilty by reason of insanity, the Court followed existing law; and in ordering appellee committed to St. Elizabeths Hospital, the Court obeyed the mandate of §301(d).[23]

The government's mechanistic interpretation suggested the possibility of the transformation of a prison into a hospital by the painting of the legend "hospital" upon the guarded portals of the prison building.

Inevitably it called for the rejoinder on behalf of Frederick Lynch that a loss of liberty was a loss of liberty, whatever the auspices under which it was inflicted. It also led me to inquire in my brief on appeal as to whether the facilities at St. Elizabeths Hospital were indeed "therapeutic" and to raise the question as to whether St. Elizabeths Hospital was in fact "a fit place for human habitation." A well-known local office-holder telephoned me almost immediately to express consternation at the attack on St. Elizabeths Hospital.

A flurry of publicity following the filing of the brief resulted in a newspaper investigation of conditions at St. Elizabeths Hospital. The investigation provided a picture typical

---

[23] *Id.,* at 25-26.

of the public mental hospital system[24] with which responsible investigators have long been acquainted.[25]

On January 26, 1961, the United States Court of Appeals reversed the District Court order and sustained the commitment of Frederick Lynch by the Municipal Court as a proper exercise of judicial discretion.

In an action without precedent in the nation, the United States Court of Appeals for the District of Columbia Circuit held:

> 1. That a defendant could be validly denied the right of entering a guilty plea to a misdemeanor even though it was conceded that he was mentally competent to participate in the proceeding against him and there was no question of coercion or undue influence, and even though defendant was effectively assisted by counsel who advised the entry of a guilty plea;
> 2. that an insanity defense could be thrust upon the defendant by either court or prosecution upon the basis of a history of some mental illness; and
> 3. that upon acquittal by reason of insanity upon the basis of a reasonable doubt as to defendant's mental health as of the time of the misdemeanor in question, the defendant was properly subject to indefinite confinement in a lunatic asylum without any hearing as to his then existing mental state.

---

[24] "An inscribed stone is imbedded in the threshold of a building at St. Elizabeths Hospital—home to some 7000 of the mentally sick.

It reads: Built, 1853-54; repaired, 1872.

One of the building's crowded men's wards is a kind of all-purpose room used for sleeping, eating and watching TV. Some of the patients pace it among a profusion of tables, beds, and benches. Others are frozen into a tableau; their eyes closed in almost endless sleep or focused on the seventeen-inch screen.

The only bath is a shower with leaky joints bound by rags which fail to keep the water from squirting into the center of the room where it forms a puddle.

The walls are heavy with layers of paint, which peel and buckle like paper. The human odors have so permeated the century-old woodwork that they defy the strongest of modern detergents." Washington Post and Herald, November 27, 1960, at A-1.

[25] *See, e.g.,* A. DEUTSCH, THE SHAME OF THE STATES (1948).

It declared that the case law of the District of Columbia established "almost a positive duty on the part of . . . [a trial judge] not to impose a criminal sentence on a mentally ill person."[26] It went on to explain that hospitalization of such a mentally ill person pursuant to District of Columbia law was "remedial and that its limitations . . . were determined by the condition to be treated," and concluded that "now that . . . [Frederick Lynch] has received treatment he is well on his way to unconditional release without the probability of repeat offenses."[27]

Three dissenters on the court declared that Frederick Lynch and his counsel "were . . . confronted with a serious situation in the Municipal Court, and the record does not show that they were given reasonable opportunity to cope with it by showing . . . [Frederick Lynch] was not of unsound mind when the checks were cashed." They went on to assert that "in the absence of that opportunity there could be no valid finding that he was not guilty by reason of insanity."[28]

They based their dissent, however, in large part on the assumption that the dangerousness capable of barring the release of Frederick Lynch under D.C. Code Ann. §301(e) (1961) of the Criminal Commitment Law was not the dangerousness of any unlawful conduct, however minor, but a dangerousness covering "the idea of physical danger to persons and, perhaps, to property."

Shortly before this decision of the Court of Appeals was handed down, Frederick Lynch had been given a "conditional release" from St. Elizabeths Hospital. He appeared, at that time, shunned by many of his erstwhile friends or acquaintances. He was also unable to secure employment commensurate with his ability and experience. He made several attempts to visit neighbors in the exclusive and

---

[26] Overholser v. Lynch, 288 F.2d 388, 393 (D.C. Cir. 1961).
[27] *Id.* at 394.
[28] *Id.,* at 395.

fashionable neighborhood in which he had once resided. One such neighbor telephoned to inform me of these events and to advise me to take every step within my means to keep my client from his doorstep. The intimation was inescapable that the police would be called in if I were not effective.

Once every three weeks Frederick Lynch was required to report to a medical officer at St. Elizabeths Hospital.

Further personal difficulties in his life coincided with a growing feeling of despair and apparent deterioration in his circumstances.

The sanguine prediction made by the majority of the Court of Appeals that "now ... that Frederick Lynch has received treatment he is well on the way to unconditional release without the probability of repeat offenses" was not borne out by subsequent events. Several relatively minor worthless checks, drawn upon his own account, appear to have been made out by Frederick Lynch as his condition deteriorated. His conditional release was revoked on April 7, 1961, on the strength of the original Municipal Court Order which had been upheld by the Court of Appeals.[29]

A petition for *certiorari* was filed with the Supreme Court and *certiorari* was granted on June 19, 1961.

The petitioner's brief, filed thereafter, claimed a violation of due process of law as well as the circumvention of the civil commitment law of the District of Columbia. It further complained of the denial of "medical due process" as a result of the prevailing conditions at St. Elizabeths Hospital. The argument I advanced was that the deprivation of liberty and reputation inflicted upon the petitioner was compounded by the fact that his restoration to society was dependent primarily upon the almost unlimited discretion of an overburdened hospital staff, devoid of adequate therapeutic and diagnostic resources, and that no commitment to a mental

---

[29] *See* United States v. Lynch, U.S. 7736-59 and U.S. 7737-59 in the Municipal Court for the District of Columbia.

institution could be deemed constitutionally justifiable save upon the assumption that the person so committed would receive adequate psychiatric treatment and rehabilitation and that such treatment was denied to Frederick Lynch.

The American Civil Liberties Union, hitherto a sponsor of this case, filed an independent amicus brief, urging the reversal of the judgment of the Court of Appeals. It relied in part on the due process clause but strongly suggested the avoidance by the Supreme Court of the constitutional issues by reliance upon statutory interpretation.

On May 21, 1962, the Supreme Court held Frederick Lynch's commitment by the Municipal Court to be null and void. It reversed the judgment of the Court of Appeals and remanded the case to the District Court. Speaking for the majority, Justice Harlan declared that it was unnecessary to consider the "constitutional claims" raised by the petitioner and proceeded to announce that the Supreme Court "read §24-301(d) as applicable only to a defendant acquitted on the ground of insanity, who affirmatively relied upon a defense of insanity and not to one, like the petitioner who has maintained that he was mentally responsible when the alleged offense was committed.[30] He further explained that §24-301(d) could not be construed as "requiring a Court, without further proceedings, automatically to commit a defendant, who, as in the present case, has competently and advisedly not tendered a defense of insanity to the crime charged and has not been found incompetent at the time of commitment. . . .[31] He concluded that "it was not Congress' purpose to make a commitment compulsory, when as here an accused disclaims reliance on a defense of mental irresponsibility."[32]

In a word, Frederick Lynch was held entitled to his freedom on the basis of the record before the Supreme Court.

---

[30] 369 U.S. 705, 710 (1962).
[31] *Id.* at 711.
[32] *Id.* at 719.

Whether as part of the holding or as an explanation thereof, Justice Harlan went on to declare:

> This does not mean, of course, that a criminal defendant has an absolute right to have his guilty plea accepted by the Court. As provided in Rule 11 Fed. Rules Crim. Proc. and Rule 9, D.C. Munic. Ct. Crim. Rules, the trial judge may refuse to accept such a plea and enter a plea of not guilty on behalf of the accused. We decide in this case only that, if this is done, and the defendant, despite his own assertion of sanity, is found not guilty by reason of insanity, §24-301(d) does not apply. If commitment is then considered warranted, it must be accomplished by resorting to §24-301(a) or by recourse to the civil commitment provisions in Title 21 of the D.C. Code.[33]

Justice Harlan, however, did not stop at this but suggested the possible use of D.C. Code Ann. § 24-301(a) as a basis for commitment of an individual after his acquittal by reason of insanity over his protest.

Section 24-301(a) was interpreted by Justice Harlan, in this context, as providing:

> a procedure for confining an accused who, though found competent to stand trial, is nonetheless committable as a person of unsound mind. That section permits the trial judge to act prior to the imposition of sentence or prior to the expiration of any period of probation, if he has reason to believe that the accused is of unsound mind *or* is mentally incompetent so as to be unable to understand the proceedings against him. . . . The statute provides for a preliminary examination by a hospital staff, and then if the court shall find the accused to be then of unsound mind or mentally incompetent to stand trial, the Court shall order the accused confined to a hospital for the mentally ill. . . . This inquiry, therefore, is not limited to the accused's competence to stand trial; the judge may consider as well, whether the accused is presently committable as a person of unsound mind. Since this inquiry may be undertaken at any time prior to the imposition of sentence, it appears to be as available after the jury returns a verdict of not guilty by reason of insanity as before trial.[34]

---

[33] *Id.* at 719-21. D.C. CODE ANN. §24-301(a) (1961) provides for commitment in language tending to confuse the issue of sanity in the abstract and that of competency to stand trial.

[34] *Id.* at 718-19.

Justice Clark dissented, asserting that the decision in Lynch undermined Congress' "humanitarian purpose of affording hospitalization for those in need of treatment."[35]

The question arises as to what the impact of the Supreme Court opinion has been upon commitment practices in the District of Columbia.

A short answer is that it has been productive of confusion and has proven an incentive to further experimentation with statutory commitment provisions as a substitute for more conventional forms of dragnet law.[36]

---

[35] Lynch v. Overholser, *supra,* at 721 (1962).

[36] The holding, if holding it was, that an individual forcibly acquitted by reason of insanity, over his protest could be subjected to confinement after a §301(a) hearing seemed to put the clock back in the District of Columbia to the days preceding Williams v. Overholser, 259 F.2d 175 (D.C. Cir. 1958). Moreover, in acting as it did the Supreme Court seemed unaware of the Williams decision of 1958. For in 1958 the Court of Appeals held in Williams v. Overholser, *supra,* that the criminal commitment power of the trial court pursuant to §24-301(a) was limited to cases involving lack of competency to stand trial. The specific interpretation of §24-301(a) made by the Court of Appeals for the District of Columbia Circuit was that the "purpose" of §24-301 was "simply to prescribe the procedure for determining whether an accused person can understand the proceedings against him and properly assist in his defense, and to provide for his confinement in a hospital instead of a jail until he can." Williams v. Overholser, *supra* at 177.

The tortured statutory interpretation of the Supreme Court suggests the obvious. Acting desperately to avoid an adjudication of constitutional claims, the Supreme Court proceeded to squeeze the complex and voluminous issues of the case into a statutory framework which can only be regarded as a product of judicial sleight of hand.

Senator Ervin, Chairman of the Senate Subcommittee on Constitutional Rights, commenting upon the oversight of the *Williams* case by the Supreme Court in its interpretation of the D.C. Commitment Law in the Lynch case declared:

"There is some consolation to some of us that even justices of the Supreme Court . . . in writing an opinion can overlook a point, . . . although . . . [it] causes a slight amount of consternation about what they will do in the future . . ." *Hearings on S.935 Before the Subcommittee on Constitutional Rights of the Senate Committee on the Judiciary,* 88th Cong., 1st Sess. at 52 (1963).

Perhaps it is best to conclude that since the Supreme Court failed to indicate any awareness of the *Williams* interpretation, which thus remained

(Footnote continued on next page.)

Finally, what about Frederick Lynch in the wake of the Supreme Court decision?

Shortly before the Supreme Court decision of his case, Frederich Lynch wrote from St. Elizabeths:

> Frankly, the conditions here are almost more than anyone can bear . . . the monotony—seventy-eight cents per day per patient food budget, no laundry, and above all no treatment. This hospital . . . is a human warehouse . . .
> Even if the Court does rule in my favor, it is kind of a case where the operation was a success but the patient died.[37]

Frederick Lynch was right. Far from assuring his release, the Supreme Court's decision of his case precipitated active consideration by the office of the public prosecutor of further commitment proceedings against him.[38]

A local newspaper noted:

> the Government had its fingers crossed in the Lynch case, because for a while it appeared that he might not be sick enough to qualify for a civil commitment.[39]

Still upon the premises of St. Elizabeths Hospital, still without treatment worthy of the name, still without hope of early release, and still the target of legal proceedings, Frederick Lynch committed suicide.[40]

---

formally unrepudiated, and since the issue before the Supreme Court was solely that of due process and the circumvention of the civil commitment law, the language of the Supreme Court relative to §301(a) could and should be viewed as mere dictum.

Significantly, in Cameron v. Mullen, 387 F.2d 193 (D.C. Cir. 1967), the Court of Appeals held that where an individual had been acquitted by reason of insanity over his objection, he was entitled to a hearing embodying substantially the procedural safeguards of civil commitment before commitment could take place.

[37] Letter to author dated January 22, 1962.

[38] Disposed initially to proceed under §24-301(a), the prosecutor's office subsequently indicated that it was preparing to proceed under the Civil Commitment Law.

[39] Washington Evening Star, August 24, 1962, at B-2.

[40] A news item, dated August 24, 1962, in the local press reported the denouément in the strange case of Frederick Lynch: "Frederick C. Lynch,
(Footnote continued on next page.)

Dr. Thomas Szasz observed:

> The Government could now uncross its fingers. Frederick Lynch, the bad-check passer, was no longer stalking the streets of Washington.[41]

---

who charged an insanity defense was forced upon him in a Municipal Court trial, yesterday threw himself under the wheels of a slow-moving truck on the grounds of St. Elizabeths Hospital, police said. The apparent suicide of the forty-five-year-old Air Force Lieutenant Colonel came on the eve of a new court hearing today in which the Government, which lost the case before the Supreme Court, sought a civil hospital commitment . . ." Washington Evening Star, August 24, 1962, at B-2.

[41] T. S. SZASZ, PSYCHIATRIC JUSTICE, 234 (1965).

Chapter V

THE QUEST FOR THE IMPARTIAL PSYCHIATRIC EXPERT: REALITY AND ILLUSION IN THE INSANITY DEFENSE

The case of John Bradley[1] is presented as a sort of *whodunnit*. The detection concerns not the discovery of the "murderer," but instead the discovery of the legal and/or psychiatric technique which seemed productive of substantial justice. On this score, there may well be differences of opinion. Certainly the psychiatrists and the lawyers differed drastically as to what accounted for the outcome of the case. This is what transpired, as I saw it.

A "Murderer" is Apprehended

John Bradley, twenty years old and a Junior at a university in Washington, D.C. was arrested on Tuesday, April 26, 1960.

At approximately 8:50 P.M. of that day an automobile pulled abreast of the firehouse on Wisconsin Avenue at Warren Street, N.W. in the City of Washington. John Bradley who drove the car jumped out and stood at the door. As the first fireman approached him, he said:

"Somebody please help, I've just killed my girl."

---

[1] A pseudonym has been substituted for the defendant's real name, therefore no attempt is made to support any colloquies by reference to the actual transcripts.

Fire Lieutenant Eugene Currier recalled:

"I took one look in the car and called the police. She was a pretty girl. The boy was just standing there shaking and holding his head."

At 8:56 P.M., a police car cruising approximately one block away, received a call for assistance from the firehouse. The police officers who arrived upon the scene within minutes were told by firemen that a woman "sitting on the front seat, with her head up against the door" appeared to be dead, because they "couldn't get any pulse" and that "that man over there at the fender said he stabbed her."

A police officer who approached John Bradley heard him "mumbling something" over a period of approximately two minutes.

After a short lapse of time, John turned upon the police officer who was searching him and said:

"I did it, I did it, love is a funny thing."

When the car was searched, a blood-stained knife was found beside the lifeless body.

John was taken to the No. 8 precinct station where he was charged with homicide.

His police interrogation began at the police station.

Detective Sergeant Arthur L. Weber described John Bradley as "nervous and upset and . . . crying and sobbing, beating his right leg with his fist."

"In between these sobs" John responded to the questioning by Sergeant Weber and others.

Sergeant Weber recounted:

> I asked him what had happened; and he told me that he had known Jane for about eight months, ever since he had gone to . . . [the] university in September of 1959; and that they had talked about getting married; that he was very much in love with her.
>
> He said that about Easter time, things began to change, and that she was going out with other boys, and that when she would see him, she would tease him about this; and that he had tried to get

... back [a ring he had given her], but she wouldn't give it back to him.

He said that about 7 P.M. that evening, that was April 26, he had a date with ... [Jane] and that he picked her up at Hughes Hall, where she lived on the campus of [the] ... university. They drove in his car around the northwest section of the city, and they went out to Bethesda to a restaurant named Tops, where they had a milkshake. They left the restaurant, and still riding around in the northwest section, said she was very bitchy. If he wanted to go one way, she wanted him to go another way.

So he said that he always got her home on time, so he went back to ... [the] university and parked on a parking lot next to a tennis court, which was adjacent to Hughes Hall; that she sat there for a few minutes; and that he told her that there was something under the front seat; and that she leaned forward to look under the front seat; and he pulled this knife and stabbed her.

He said that as soon as he had stabbed her, he saw that she was hurt, he thought of getting first aid for her. When he thought of first aid, he thought of firemen. So that he drove down to Wisconsin Avenue, to the firehouse, and tried to get someone to help him with her.

John was asked among other things to show the police where the stabbing had taken place and he obliged by getting into the "cruiser" and directing the police to a parking lot near the university campus. As he was being driven back to No. 8, he was asked as to where he had purchased the knife and he told the police that it was in a store on Wisconsin Avenue. He then said that long before the events that had led to his arrest

he had tried to get help. He'd gone to two people for help and he mentioned one of them, ... it was a Bess Ninaj of the Washington Sanitarium. He said that he ... told this lady that he had an impulse to kill this girl and she talked him out of it.

He further told the police that he had "talked to a ... counselor at the university ..." During much of his interrogation at No. 8 he would lower his voice, put his head in his hands and lapse into silence. "His face was red, flushed."

Shortly after his arrival at No. 8, the police called a member of the United States Attorney's office who advised them "that the next morning was time enough for arraignment."

About 10:00 P.M., John was taken to the homicide squad. The office of the homicide squad is across the street from the United States District Court Building. His interrogation at the homicide squad began sometime after midnight. The usual written statement admitting guilt was secured. Throughout this time John was held incommunicado.

John's arraignment was held about 9:00 A.M. April 27 1960.[2]

The coroner's inquest followed on April 29, 1960. Only then was John formally represented by counsel. Mr. Myron Ehrlich had been retained by the parents. (He subsequently requested that I join him as co-counsel in the case.) The inquest heard testimony concerning the cause of death. Firemen and police officers also testified about John's agitated state at the time of his arrest and for some time after that.

John followed the testimony against him without apparent difficulty. He was described by newspaper reporters who were present as presenting a "face flushed and contorted by grief and anxiety" and as "alternately wringing his hands

---

[2] Rule 5(a), F.R.Cr.P. provided as follows:

"An officer making an arrest under a warrant issued upon a complaint or any person making an arrest without a warrant shall take the arrested person *without unnecessary delay* before the nearest available commissioner or before any other nearby officer empowered to commit persons charged with offenses against the laws of the United States." (Emphasis supplied).

The Supreme Court has declared such safeguards to be essential "against the misuse of the law enforcement process." McNabb v. United States, 318 U.S. 332 (1943); Upshaw v. United States, 335 U.S. 410 (1948).

The rule is specifically designed to prevent prolonged or intensive interrogation for the purpose of securing damaging statements to be used against the accused. See, e.g., Goldsmith v. United States, 277 F.2d 335 (D.C. Cir. 1960).

and running them through his closecropped blond hair . . ."[3]

The Coroner's Jury declared John Bradley responsible for the death of Jane and held him for the action of the Grand Jury. Preparation of the defense now began in earnest.

His two lawyers viewed insanity as perhaps the most plausible defense under the circumstances. The problem was one of selecting a psychiatric team which could be viewed as scientifically reliable and effective within the courtroom.

A PSYCHIATRIC TEAM IS SELECTED BY THE DEFENSE

Myron Ehrlich had at first retained the services of the late Dr. Manfred Guttmacher of Baltimore.

On May 6, 1960, Dr. Guttmacher, accompanied by Dr. Leonard H. Ainsworth, a psychologist, conducted a psychiatric interview of several hours' duration of John Bradley in the District Jail. Dr. Ainsworth administered standard psychological tests.

Dr. Guttmacher described his patient as a person with "modest intellectual endowment" who was suffering from "profound feelings of inadequacy and a very marked obsessive-compulsive personality makeup." He went on to state, however, that he did not believe that one could assert that he was psychotic. He added that the patient was "extremely vulnerable psychiatrically and might well be given to what Dr. Karl Menninger called 'periods of episodic dyscontrol' which are essentially psychotic in nature."

He concluded as follows:

> Whether this comes within the confines of mental disease as laid down in the Durham decision is a moot question and one that will have to be determined by the court.
> This Examiner would like to have the benefit of all of the

---

[3] A Washington newspaper in 1960.

> data which defense counsel is able to collect about this patient's past behavior, particularly during the period since he has been at the . . . university.
>
> He also feels at this time that it will probably be necessary for him to hear the evidence at the trial before reaching a final decision in regard to the patient's responsibility.[4]

Dr. Guttmacher's report was impressively comprehensive in covering the life history of the boy in substantial detail.

I interviewed John Bradley on approximately two occasions shortly after my entry into the case.

I was struck by his apparent outward normalcy, friendliness and cooperation, and concluded that it would be wise to proceed upon the assumption that there was a substantial possibility that psychiatric examination would uncover only evidence of nonpsychotic mental disorder. It seemed urgent therefore that the defense secure psychiatric experts predisposed to view the victims of psychoneuroses and personality disorders as mentally ill.

Dr. Guttmacher, who talked with me over the telephone at that time, inquired as to whether an obsessive-compulsive personality could be validly regarded as within the purview of mental illness under the *Durham* rule.

Although I had high regard for Dr. Guttmacher as a leader in his profession, as well as for the thoroughness of his psychiatric study of the case, I suggested that we secure the services of psychoanalysts more willing to regard a neurotic character structure as within the purview of mental or emotional illness.

For better or worse, I was biased in favor of the employment of psychoanalytic techniques in the study of our client.

My predispositions as well as those of the Court of Appeals, as I understood them from a reading of *Carter v. United States,* seemed to be to regard the psychoanalyst as preeminently qualified to conduct such a study.[5]

---

[4] Report to Counsel, dated May 10, 1960.
[5] *See* Carter v. United States, 252 F.2d 608, 617 (D.C. Cir. 1957).

During the second week of May, 1960, Dr. Leon Salzman, a senior psychiatrist of the Washington School of Psychiatry and Dr. Edward Sachar, a young psychiatrist who had recently joined the staff of the Walter Reed Army Medical Center, were requested by us to conduct a systematic study of the patient with a view to securing an explanation of his condition and its dynamics. They commenced their study before the end of May. Both doctors at that time were asked to establish as intensive a professional relationship with the patient as they deemed feasible and helpful.

Both saw the patient for approximately two sessions a week.

Dr. Salzman's initial reactions were primarily those of academic interest in what he described as an "obsessive" and/or "schizoid" state. At times a note of wry amusement would creep into his comments on his patient as, for example, when he said that he had just seen Bradley and that Bradley "in his strange schizoid way" was happily assuming that he was in no immediate danger and that all would be well.

Dr. Sachar communicated a feeling for what he saw as the inner torment of the boy.

When I saw John in the jail about the end of the month he inquired about Dr. Sachar and declared that he had found it easier to talk to him than to any other doctor and that he wished that he could see him more frequently.

At about this time, Dr. Salzman indicated that he wished to proceed with his study of this case on his own. He added that during his summer vacation he would wish to turn the case over temporarily to Dr. Paul Chodoff, also of the Washington School of Psychiatry.

Dr. Sachar told me almost simultaneously that Dr. Salzman did not seem to welcome any conferences with him and that he therefore felt that he should leave the case.

I acquiesced in Dr. Sachar's resignation and accepted Dr. Salzman's association with Dr. Chodoff.

THE FIRST CLASH BETWEEN DEFENSE AND PROSECUTION

As was to be expected, the prosecution was at that time working to secure an indictment against John Bradley for murder in the first degree. Inevitably it had to depend on a showing of "deliberate and premeditated malice."[6]

Rumors reaching the defense during this period of preparation could not always be traced back to their source. It would be dishonest to assert that they were wholly disregarded. We had been informed that a senior psychiatrist at St. Elizabeths Hospital had, on the basis of either newspaper coverage or data furnished to him by the United States Attorney's office, stated to a professional colleague that it appeared clear that Bradley's act was a product of premeditation and deliberation. This assumed even more serious significance when we heard that Miss Bess Ninaj, a religious counselor at the Washington Sanitarium to whom John had confided about "an impulse to kill" was subpoenaed to testify before the Grand Jury.

On May 20, 1960, the prosecution moved before Chief Judge Letts for a mental examination of John Bradley by psychiatrists of its selection and it further moved to compel a recalcitrant, Miss Bess Ninaj, to testify as to the disclosures made to her, as a religious counselor, by John Bradley during his relationship with the deceased. The motion papers asserted that the United States Attorney's office had been informed by Mr. Ehrlich that he had retained Dr. Guttmacher to conduct a mental examination of his client, that Mr. Ehrlich had advised the United States Attorney's office that "he could not acquiesce in . . . [a] proposed examination by . . . [a] psychiatrist to be selected by the government" and that Miss Bess Ninaj had refused

---

[6] D.C. CODE, ANN. §22-2401 provides as follows:
"Whoever, being of sound memory and discretion, kills another purposely, either of deliberate and premeditated malice or by means of poison . . . is guilty of murder in the first degree."

to answer questions before the Grand Jury under a claim of the penitent-clergyman privilege.

Mr. Smithson of the United States Attorney's office argued that the court should take judicial notice of the fact that the government psychiatrists had been saying

> that the longer you wait from the time of the act to the time . . . [the psychiatrists] have a chance to look at . . . [a defendant], the more difficult [it is] for them to give a valid, lucid, clearly understood explanation of what, if any, condition they might find.

Mr. Smithson concluded by stating:

> I see nothing to be harmful to the defendant by this practice, unless it is to be said that the defendant has a right to utilize a defense of insanity and to forestall the government from carrying its burden under the statute of offering some evidence and to forestall it by this means, by refusing to let a government psychiatrist talk to this defendant or examine him. I do not believe that the Court of Appeals in any of the decisions has ever gone so far as to say that a defendant may utilize such a defense and forbid, by such a maneuver, the government, in opposing this motion.

The defense pointed out that § 24-301(a) of the District of Columbia Code authorized mental examinations only upon the court's own observation or on prima facie evidence submitted to the court that the accused was of unsound mind or incompetent and that no such basis for a mental examination had been set forth in the government's motion.

Mr. Ehrlich went on to state:

> Now, our principal objection to have this mental examination is caused not because we have any desire to thwart the government . . . [in] examining this boy, but because we have already arranged to have this boy mentally examined and Your Honor knows as well as I know that a proper examination of an accused . . . by a qualified psychiatrist means that that psychiatrist and that person whom he is examining have to have an intimate relationship, that is, an intimate relationship between doctor and patient which excludes the intervention of other persons examining him, because what we are afraid of is that the intervention of all of these government psychiatrists will not permit a proper

diagnosis and a prognosis of the defendant in this case by the psychiatrists whom we have asked to examine him.

Now, further, we believe that this is a case which requires an examination by competent psychoanalysts, and Mr. Smithson knows and I know and Your Honor knows that St. Elizabeths Hospital does not have provision for psychoanalysts, . . .

Now, with all those things in mind, I am merely saying to the Court that as a matter of justice, we are entitled not to have the government doctors interfere with the examination of this boy at this time, because it would interfere with the psychiatrists whom we have retained at great expense to the boy's family, . . .

And further than that, there is no foundation in this motion for this Court or any court to order a mental examination because, first and foremost, you must allege, and he hasn't done so, what the Code says must be alleged, that he has some prima facie evidence that the accused is of unsound mind, and he hasn't alleged it, and I suggest he has not alleged it for a particular reason, which is obvious to the Court and to Mr. Smithson and to me.

I suggest to the Court for all of those reasons that Your Honor ought not to order a mental examination of this boy at this time. Now, it may well be that in the near future we may come in and consent to the mental examination being ordered of this defendant, but we are not ready to do so now.

The court, however, granted the government's motion, entering an order for the examination of John Bradley by Dr. William G. Cushard, a psychiatrist of the government's selection.

Immediately after the disposition of this matter, Mr. Stevas, the Assistant United States Attorney in charge of the presentation of the evidence in the Bradley case before the Grand Jury rose to inform the court that Miss Bess Ninaj, duly subpoenaed to testify before the Grand Jury had, upon advice of the defense, refused to testify to conversations which she had had with the defendant under the minister-penitent privilege. Mr. Stevas went on to say that these conversations were material to the Grand Jury investigation insofar as they bore "upon the defendant's state of mind, motive, [and] intent . . ." He concluded by asking the court to "direct her to answer these questions pertaining to the conversations which she had with the defendant . . . on the ground that she is not an ordained minister and that the defendant is not of her own faith. . . ."

Mr. Ehrlich's basic argument was not only that a minister-penitent privilege obtained under the circumstances but that "a communication made in reasonable confidence that it will not be disclosed and, in such circumstances that disclosure is shocking to the moral sense of the community, should not be disclosed in a judicial proceeding whether the trusted person is or is not a wife, husband, doctor, lawyer or minister."[7]

Miss Bess Ninaj took the witness stand to testify that she was a Seventh Day Adventist and that her "entire time . . . [was] devoted to spiritual ministry with people of all denominations." She went on to assert that she believed that "[John Bradley] came to . . . [her] because . . . [she was] a religious spiritual counselor . . . [and that he] came to . . . [her] in confidence."

Cross-examination revealed that Miss Ninaj was not qualified by the rules of her church to conduct a marriage cere-

---

[7] This argument was based upon the language of Judge Edgerton in Mullen v. United States, 263 F.2d 275 (D.C.Cir. 1959):
"I think a communication made in reasonable confidence that it will not be disclosed and in such circumstances that disclosure is shocking to the moral sense of the community, should not be disclosed in a judicial proceeding, whether the trusted person is or is not a wife, husband, doctor, lawyer or minister. As Mr. Justice Holmes said of wire-tapping, 'We have to choose and for my part I think it a less evil that some criminals should escape than that the Government should play an ignoble part.'" *Id.*, at 281.

The trend of judicial opinion has been to recognize privilege within an expanding context of confidential relations.

As expressed by the New York Court of Appeals, it is "long standing public policy to encourage uninhibited communications between persons standing in a relation of confidence and trust, such as husband and wife, confessor and clergyman, or doctor and patient, attorney and client. In carrying out such a policy, the statutes are accorded a broad and liberal construction." (*dictum*) People v. Shapiro, 308 N.Y. 453, 126 N.E. 2d 559, 561-562 (1955).

For a view of the extension of the privilege to a mere investigator in the service of the Government *see* Totten v. United States, 92 U.S. 105 (1875).

mony but that she could conduct a baptismal ceremony in an emergency.

She denied that her position with the Seventh Day Adventists approximated that of a Sunday school teacher.

The court inquired as to whether she had "kept the information obtained by . . . [her] through [her] contact with the defendant [John Bradley], absolutely and truly in confidence." She replied:

"To the best of my knowledge Sir."

The court thereupon stated that "the privilege asked by this witness should be recognized and the Grand Jury is so instructed." Nonetheless, an indictment charging Bradley with murder in the first degree was returned shortly afterwards.

THE DILEMMA POSED BY THE PSYCHIATRISTS FOR THE PROSECUTION

The immediate problem facing us was whether we were to advise our client to talk to Dr. Cushard, the expert selected by the prosecution. Dr. Cushard was a Clinical Director at St. Elizabeths Hospital.

Past experience had not fostered a sense of confidence in the hospital which—if able to express an opinion concerning our client—might literally decide whether he was to live or die.

There was, it appeared to us, a substantial possibility that our client would be subjected to hostile, rather than objective psychiatric scrutiny in the course of any examination conducted by such a prosecution expert at this stage. We further believed that even objective psychiatric scrutiny by mediocre members of the profession would not yield evidence conducive to a finding of mental disorder. In the words of one of the defense psychiatrists, "the boy appeared calm, rational, and entirely cooperative. . . . The initial impression that he made on the psychiatrists"—and these were the psychiatrists for the defense—"was that of a somewhat immature young man who struck out in fury when he did not get what he wanted, and thus killed his girl-friend."[8]

The subjection of our client to mental examination by a staff member of St. Elizabeths Hospital struck us, therefore, as tending toward the incrimination of our client in the sense that a limited or prosecution-oriented examination tended to the production of psychiatric data which would be used by the government to negative the insanity defense and thus secure the conviction of our client on a charge of murder.[9]

We further believed that Dr. Salzman's program of psychodynamic exploration might be disrupted by third party intervention.

It was our joint judgment, therefore, that whatever doubts existed concerning the intervention of the St. Elizabeths staff in a situation in which a life was so immediately at stake should be resolved against the staff in favor of the individual defendant. Regardless of whether or not the case against any member of the St. Elizabeths Hospital could be documented by substantial evidence, the voice of caution impelled us to advise our client that he refuse to talk with any person not directly introduced to him by his counsel.

I informed John Bradley that his interests were most likely to be safeguarded by not entering into any conversation with Dr. Cushard.

On May 31, 1960, the United States Attorney's Office received the following letter from Dr. Cushard.

---

[8] Salzman, *Psychiatric Interviews as Evidence,* 30 GEO. WASH. L. REV. 853, 868 (1962).

[9] However indirectly, submission of the defendant to psychiatric examination was susceptible to the development of psychiatric data capable of being used to defeat the insanity defense and hence to exact the forfeiture of the defendant's life upon his trial for murder. In other words, a defendant cooperating with either hostile or skeptical psychiatrists literally cooperated in his own undoing. *See, e.g.,* Douglas, J., dissenting, in Breithaupt v. Abram, 352 U.S. 432, 443 (1957).

Honorable Oliver Gasch
United States Attorney
for the District of Columbia
Washington, D.C.
Attention: Mr. Frederick G. Smithson
Assistant United States Attorney

Dear Mr. Gasch:

In accordance with the request of Mr. Frederick G. Smithson, Assistant United States Attorney, and by authority of a Court Order signed by Judge Letts of the United States District Court for the District of Columbia, I went to the District of Columbia Jail on May 29, 1960 at 8:50 A.M. to examine Mr. John . . . [Bradley] (G.J. No. XX . . .) I saw Mr. . . . [Bradley] in the hospital section of the D.C. Jail, third floor, and advised him that I was there to perform a psychiatric examination on a Court Order. He told me that he had been advised by his lawyer not to talk to anyone. I told him that since he had been so advised by counsel I, of course, accepted his decision not to be examined.

I am sorry that I was unable to examine Mr. . . . [Bradley] and make a determination of his mental condition.

Sincerely yours,
/s/ William G. Cushard
William G. Cushard, M.D.

On June 3, 1960, the prosecution filed a motion for mental examination of the defendant to be conducted at St. Elizabeths Hospital pursuant to §24-301(a) of the District of Columbia Code.

The motion did not advert to any *prima facie* evidence of lack of mental competency of the defendant to stand trial beyond that presented by the following allegations:

The United States Attorney's Office has been reliably informed that the defendant, John . . . [Bradley], has been examined by the following doctors on the dates and at the approximate times indicated:
1. On May 6, 1960, from 9:05 A.M. to 11:50 A.M., by Dr. Manfred Guttmacher, a psychiatrist from Baltimore, Maryland.
2. On May 6, 1960, from 9:05 A.M. to 12:40 P.M. by Dr. L.H. Ainsworth, a psychologist.
3. On May 22, 1960, from 1:55 P.M. to 4:20 P.M. by Dr. Edward Sachar, a psychiatrist from Walter Reed Hospital.
4. On May 28, 1960, from 11:08 A.M. to 1:20 P.M., by Dr. Leon Salzman, a psychiatrist.

In a written opposition to the motion for mental examination, we asserted:

> Dr. Salzman . . . [claims] that transfer of the defendant to St. Elizabeths Hospital before the completion of the diagnostic program planned for defendant under the Doctor's supervision at the District of Columbia Jail will disrupt the investigation which is now in progress and will jeopardize the adequate completion of the Doctor's professional work in this case. Counsel for defendant have established an intensive program of psychiatric and psychoanalytic investigation involving at least four highly trained medical specialists at great expense to the family of the defendant, and the transfer of the defendant to St. Elizabeths Hospital will, as shown by Doctor Salzman's affidavit attached hereto, disrupt the presently existing diagnostic program, established by the defense, jeopardize the medical preparation of defendant's case, and hence inevitably interfere with the defendant's right to a fair trial as well as of effective assistance of counsel, which inevitably hinges upon adequate expert assistance in preparation in this case.

Dr. Salzman, in an affidavit in support of our opposition asserted as follows:

> I have personally examined the defendant in this case and am in charge of all medical evaluation concerning the defendant's mental state as of the time of the crime charged in the indictment at the request of the defendant's counsel. The series of examinations undertaken by me and under my supervision, and still far from completion at this date, are designed to provide a view in depth of the defendant's condition, whatever its character, at the time of the alleged crime, i.e. how it arose, developed and affected the defendant's mental and emotional processes. It is my professional opinion that such examinations in depth can be adequately conducted only by intensive psychoanalytic techniques. These techniques have been utilized in carrying out the examinations so far and will continue in the future.
> It is also my professional opinion that the series of psychoanalytic interviews contemplated for the defendant, demand an atmosphere of intimacy and confidentiality between patient and doctor for successful results on both the therapeutic level as well as in the appraisal of the dynamic elements involved in resolving the issue of insanity at the time of the alleged crime. Such an atmosphere, in my professional opinion, would definitely suffer from the intervention of third parties outside the psychoanalytical relationship.

> It is my further professional opinion that transfer of the defendant to St. Elizabeths Hospital before the completion of the diagnostic and psychotherapeutic program planned for him under my supervision at the District Jail will disrupt the investigation which is now in progress and jeopardize the adequate completion of my professional work in this case, as described, for the reasons stated above.

At the hearing of the motion on June 20, 1960, Mr. Ehrlich further pointed to inadequacies of St. Elizabeths Hospital in the conduct of an examination in depth and offered to submit our client without any delay to examination by appropriately trained psychiatrists selected by the chairmen of the Departments of Psychiatry of Georgetown and George Washington University Medical Schools and the Director of the National Institute of Mental Health.

Mr. Ehrlich stated at that time that on completion of preliminary studies by our doctors our client would be made available to the examination of medical experts of the prosecution's choosing even at St. Elizabeths Hospital. When the court inquired as to how much time that would take, Mr. Ehrlich turned to me for information and I stated it would be a minimum of six to eight weeks.

The District Court bypassed both these offers and granted the motion of the government.

John Bradley was ordered transferred to St. Elizabeths Hospital for a period not to exceed ninety days to enable the staff of that hospital to determine whether he was "presently so mentally incompetent as to be unable to understand the proceedings against him" and whether "at the time of the alleged criminal offense, committed on or about April 26, 1960, [he] was suffering from a mental disease or defect, and if so, whether his criminal act was the product of his mental condition. . . ."

The order contained the further stipulation "that the Superintendent of St. Elizabeths Hospital . . . [should] permit Dr. Paul Chodoff, Dr. Leon Salzman, Dr. Edward Sachar, Dr. Manfred Guttmacher, and two additional psychiatrists to be designated by Dr. Salzman, to conduct such examinations of the defendant as they require[d] for the purpose of their determination, at the mutual convenience of the physicians named above, and of the staff of St. Elizabeths Hospital..."

We challenged this order by a petition for a writ of prohibition in the Court of Appeals.

Our reasons were varied.

We believed, of course, that there was a possibility that the Court Order directing the examination of our client in a hostile environment would be set aside. Since, moreover, the doctors of St. Elizabeths had committed themselves to the view that reliability of psychiatric determinations concerning mental states as of a past date was directly proportioned to the proximity in time of such examination to the date of the alleged crime,[10] we further believed that

---

[10] The view of St. Elizabeths Hospital as to the importance of early psychiatric examination was clearly stated by its superintendent, Dr. Winfred Overholser, in the following letter regarding another case:

"May 25, 1960
"Dear Mr. Arens:

The following information is submitted in response to your letter of May 23, 1960, regarding John A. Gearhart.

It is true that we were unable to form an opinion as to the presence, or absence, of mental disease in this patient during the period April to August, 1958, because it would have meant projecting backward in time for eighteen to twenty-two months prior to the time that we first had an opportunity to examine him. Your inquiry is intimately related to a problem which some of our physicians, who are involved in forensic psychiatric work, have been trying to impress on all concerned: that in order to form opinions regarding the mental condition of patients (opinions having any reasonable basis), it is necessary in the great majority of cases to have the opportunity to examine the patient just as soon as possible after the commission of the crime. If the examination can be done within twenty-four to forty-eight hours, firm opinions can be formed in most cases. With the passage of each additional day, the probability of forming such opinions decreases; and, after a month or so has elapsed we get progressively more and more into the realm of speculation. Since courts are not interested in speculations it is, in many cases, impossible to form or render opinions as time passes. If psychiatrists are to be of
(Footnote continued on next page.)

every day's delay was a day gained in favor of the defendant. Obviously, therefore, much was to be gained from delaying the transfer of our client to that hostile environment. There was, beyond this, a third compelling reason for our action. In setting forth before the Court of Appeals the elaborate program for the psychoanalytic exploration of our client's mental state in detail, in disclosing the names of leading members of the psychiatric profession who were to participate in it, in stressing our efforts to meet the standards set by the Court of Appeals in the *Carter* case, and finally in pointing to the inability of St. Elizabeths Hospital to meet those self-same standards, we served notice upon St. Elizabeths of the diagnostic complexity of the case, the need for maximal care in its assessment and finally of the presence of élite psychiatrists who would regard an inadequate diagnostic work-up by its staff as a disservice to its profession.

Our chief contention was highlighted in these terms:

> Interference with the psychoanalytic investigation conducted under the supervision of Dr. Salzman, therefore, will eliminate the opportunity to prepare a defense, to which the petitioner has a constitutional right. The elimination of such opportunity . . . is not remediable upon appeal because the point reached at this time in the petitioner's psychoanalytic exploration is not likely to be recaptured, in the light of available medical knowledge, and a psychoanalytic exploration *de novo* might and probably would be fatally handicapped.

We then proceeded to refer to the inadequacies of the facilities of the John Howard Pavilion of the St. Elizabeths Hospital for the conduct of psychiatric examinations.

---

any considerable value to the courts in this type of case, it seems imperative that some legal way of obtaining prompt examination be devised.

           "Sincerely yours,
           /s/ Winfred Overholser
           Winfred Overholser, M.D.
           Superintendent"

We asserted as follows:

> It is a fact, attested by the latest publication of the members and fellows of the American Psychiatric Association, that none of the "psychiatrists" at the John Howard Pavilion at St. Elizabeths Hospital has passed the examination of the American Board of Neurology and Psychiatry, and that none has been certified by that Board as a qualified psychiatric practitioner . . .

Argument on the petition was heard by an interested panel of the Court of Appeals on June 23, 1960.

Without notice to his counsel and without awaiting the decision of the Court of Appeals, the Marshal's office, however, moved Bradley into St. Elizabeths Hospital upon the morning of the argument.

As had been expected, the Court of Appeals denied the writ.

Our information was, however, that the proceedings in the Court of Appeals had not passed unnoticed by the medical staff of the John Howard Pavilion of St. Elizabeths Hospital. We were informed that several St. Elizabeths physicians had expressed themselves as pained by the apparent disparagement of their professional qualifications and by the suggestion that they seemed unable to cope with subtle manifestations of psychotic psychopathology.

John Bradley, now at St. Elizabeths, refused to cooperate even to the point of removing his clothes for a physical examination.

An anguished telephone call from a St. Elizabeths physician to us resulted in our telling John that he could submit to the physical examination demanded by the staff doctors.

On July 14, 1960, the Superintendent of St. Elizabeths Hospital addressed the following letter to the Clerk of the District Court:

> July 14, 1960
>
> Dear Sir:
> The attention of the Honorable Court is invited to the case of John . . . [Bradley] (Criminal Number XX). Mr. John . . .

[Bradley] was admitted to Saint Elizabeths Hospital June 23, 1960, by order of the United States District Court for the District of Columbia, for a period not to exceed ninety days pursuant to the provisions of Title 24, Section 301 of the District of Columbia Code. The Order directed that the patient be examined by the psychiatric staff of Saint Elizabeths Hospital to determine (1) Whether the defendant is presently so mentally incompetent as to be unable to understand the proceedings against him or to properly assist in the preparation of his defense; and, (2) Whether the defendant at the time of the alleged criminal offense, committed on or about April 26, 1960, was suffering from a mental disease or defect and, if so, whether his criminal act was the product of his mental condition. It was further ordered that the Superintendent of Saint Elizabeths Hospital permit Dr. Paul Chodoff, Dr. Leon Salzman, Dr. Edward Sachar, Dr. Manfred Guttmacher, and two additional psychiatrists to be designated by Dr. Salzman, to conduct such examinations of the defendant as they require for the purpose of their determination, at the mutual convenience of the named physicians and the staff of Saint Elizabeths Hospital.

Since his admission to Saint Elizabeths Hospital, John . . . [Bradley] has refused to be examined by the psychiatric staff of Saint Elizabeths Hospital, stating that he is taking this position on the advice of counsel. In view of the fact that we are unable to make a determination of Mr. . . . [Bradley's] mental condition as the result of his refusal to be examined on the advice of counsel, it is respectfully requested that Mr. . . . [Bradley] be removed from Saint Elizabeths Hospital to another appropriate institution to be designated by the Honorable Court.

> Sincerely yours,
> /s/ Winfred Overholser
> Winfred Overholser, M.D.
> Superintendent

On July 25, 1960, the Government filed a motion to amend the Order for mental examination in the following fashion:

ORDERED, that the defendant be and he is hereby committed to Saint Elizabeths Hospital for a period not to exceed ninety (90) days for examination by the psychiatric staff of that hospital, *and the defendant is ordered to cooperate with the psychiatric staff of said hospital* in the manner and to the extent necessary to enable the staff to comply with the previous Order of This Court, signed by Chief Judge David A. Pine, dated June 20, 1960. Such cooperation shall extend to physical, neurological, psychological and X-ray studies and psychiatric interviews but

not be limited thereto; and that after such examination a report be made to this Court as to:
1. Whether the defendant is presently so mentally incompetent as to be unable to understand the proceedings against him or to properly assist in the preparation of his defense herein; and
2. Whether the defendant, at the time of the alleged criminal offense committed on or about April 26, 1960, was suffering from a mental disease, or defect, and if so, whether his criminal act was the product of his mental condition.

The primary basis of the motion was the letter by Dr. Overholser. The motion, however, was further supported by an affidavit by Dr. David Owens of the St. Elizabeths staff, who declared:

> On June 20, 1960, an Order of the United States District Court for the District of Columbia, signed by Chief Judge David A. Pine, ordered "that the defendant be and he is hereby committed to Saint Elizabeths Hospital for a period not to exceed ninety days for examination by the psychiatric staff of that hospital and that after such examination a report be made to this Court . . ." Since his admission to Saint Elizabeths Hospital, John S. [Bradley] . . . has refused to be examined by me, as a member of the psychiatric staff of Saint Elizabeths Hospital, stating that he is taking this position on the advice of counsel. Several attempts have been made by me to conduct a mental examination of Mr. . . . [Bradley] but on each occasion he has refused to cooperate with the examination. However, it has been noted that he cooperates in ward activities, recreational activities, and in caring for his own needs. It is my firm opinion that his refusal to cooperate with the mental examination is a deliberate effort by him to avoid a mental examination by the psychiatric staff of Saint Elizabeths and is not due to a mental condition which would make cooperation impossible.

When the motion came on to be heard on September 16, 1960, before Chief Judge Pine, the prosecution argued that the defendant had frustrated a lawful order of the court, that that order should be properly enforced against him and all those connected with him and that compliance with that order would in no way result in the infringement of the defendant's privilege against self-incrimination insofar as the District Statute explicitly excluded confidential communications made by a patient to a doctor acting in his professional capacity. As expressed by Mr. Smithson for the government, the defendant should not "be allowed to play fast and loose with the government on this type of a matter, where he will cooperate, as he is doing at present with his own physicians and refusing flatly, on the advice of counsel, to cooperate with those appointed by this court, pursuant to the government's request."

The thinking of the prosecution was clearly to the effect that an insanity defense was being fabricated by unscrupulous counsel. We were told that under the circumstances of the case the "affirmative defense of insanity... shows a lack of honesty" and in point of fact "a prevarication on . . . [the defendant's] part and actually of fraud. . ."

Such was the temper in which the motion for a court order directing the defendant to cooperate with prosecution psychiatrists was argued.

Early in the argument the judge turned to the prosecutor to inquire:

> Suppose I order him to do as you pray and he still refuses. What am I going to do? How can I enforce that? . . .
> I want to know how. I cannot find him in contempt. That would not hurt him any.

Prosecuting counsel readily admitted that contempt action against the defendant would be "ridiculous."

The following colloquy ensued:

THE COURT: Do you think it wise for the Court to sign an Order it cannot enforce?
THE PROSECUTION: I think, Your Honor.—I don't know what to advise the Court other than this is what I think is in the sense of fairness and justice and equity.
THE COURT: This is not responsive to my question.
THE PROSECUTION: Yes, sir. I think Your Honor should sign

the Order for this reason: I believe Your Honor should sign the Order because he is freely and voluntarily talking to physicians, psychiatrists of his own choice as I believe Dr. Owens would be here to testify.

THE COURT: I still say that you are not responding to my question. Should the Court sign any Order that it cannot enforce?

THE PROSECUTION: Your Honor, part of this Order you could enforce . . . you can take the statement of Dr. Owens, that is, that the defendant is refusing to cooperate on advice of counsel. That is one possibility and the other, as to the defendant himself, no, there isn't much— it is a rather futile gesture as to him except the government wants to preserve this point because we would hope to offer and have accepted at the time of trial, when this issue is raised, that this was a deliberate attempt on his part to frustrate . . . the tests under Title 24-301 on insanity, [and] the Douglas and Wright decisions putting the burden on us.

THE COURT: Do you think that I could find counsel in contempt for advising their clients according to their best judgment?

THE PROSECUTION: I think, your Honor, that the point of whether or not they advise him not to comply with a Court Order, I think possibly could be done.

As I understand it this man has advised the doctor that he will not cooperate on the advice of counsel with the Court Order for an examination.

THE COURT: I just asked those questions. You are asking for an Order that apparently is unenforceable if not obeyed.

THE PROSECUTION: As to the defendant.

THE COURT: Is not that the same as to counsel?

THE PROSECUTION: I wouldn't carry it that far, no, sir.

THE COURT: Do you mean to say that when a counsel advises his client not to make any statements, exercising their honest judgment, that then the Court can find them in contempt?

THE PROSECUTION: If defense counsel advised any defendant not to comply with a lawful Court Order, I believe a citation is possible, yes, sir.
THE COURT: All right.

It was clear beyond peradventure that the prosecution was seeking a test case in which counsel would be held in contempt for advising a client to refuse to talk to government doctors.

It seemed natural under these circumstances for Mr. Ehrlich to state in response that:

> [he] came here today thinking that . . . [he] was representing a defendant but from Mr. Smithson's argument, apparently he has made Mr. Arens and . . . [Mr. Ehrlich] the defendants.

Mr. Ehrlich then went on to declare that the products of hostile psychiatric scrutiny, secured against the will of the defendant, constituted in and of themselves a violation of the rights of the defendant under the Fifth Amendment. He went on to point out that since—under the *Winn* case—[11] the determination of mental capacity by government doctors "requires adequate knowledge and a proper expert evaluation of the accused's personal history and the circumstances surrounding the crime" a coerced psychiatric examination of the kind demanded by the government clearly violated the defendant's rights:

> If a doctor can testify about the circumstances surrounding the crime, what happens to the defendant's right under the Fifth Amendment?

Indirect incrimination, moreover, was pointed out as just as hazardous as the direct variety and equally proscribed in the Constitution.

The court, however, granted the motion of the government and declared:

---

[11] Winn v. United States, 270 F.2d 326 (D.C. Cir. 1959).

I think it would be an intolerable situation if the government should be deprived of the opportunity to ascertain the truth and that being my feeling, I am going to grant the Motion.

Whether I can enforce it, if there is refusal to obey, that is something else.[12]

The first order in the history of the District of Columbia which directed a defendant charged with murder to cooperate with government psychiatrists in the assessment of his mental state, was signed by Judge Pine on September 19, 1960.

As we reviewed the progress of the case approximately one week after the entry of this District Court Order, it appeared to us that since we had succeeded in securing the unfettered period of time we had initially declared necessary for our experts, we would be harming the public image of our case if we advised our client to continue his noncooperation with the St. Elizabeths' doctors. But we at no time intended to abandon our assertion of the boy's constitutional immunity from psychiatric examination at St. Elizabeths. The presence of the Court Order constituted, in our opinion, duress which rendered any data obtained from our client by the prosecution's staff inadmissible in any court proceedings. It was our intention, therefore, in the event of adverse findings by the St. Elizabeths' staff, to object to all the St. Elizabeths' testimony as the product of

---

[12] It would seem highly doubtful, to say the least, that counsel, advising a client in good faith as to his legal rights could be subject to contempt proceedings. It is questionable in fact if counsel would not be guilty of dereliction of duty to their client in failing to warn him of the dangers of cooperation with the government physicians in this case. *See e.g.,* Galagher v. Municipal Court of Los Angeles, 31 Cal. 2d. 784, 192 P 2d 905 (1948).

Certainly it is clear beyond any doubt that advice by a lawyer to disregard a Court Order believed in good faith to be violative of statutory or constitutional law is not punishable as misconduct falling "within the category of acts which constitute contempt in open court where immediate punishment 'is necessary to prevent demoralization of the court's authority' . . . or the other types of contempt considered in Brown v. United States, 359 U.S. 41 . . ." *In Re* Green's Petition, 369 U.S. 689, 692 (1962).

coerced cooperation, violative of the privilege against self-incrimination and the due process clause of the Fifth Amendment.[13]

We thereafter informed our client that he should yield to the dictate of the court.

In October, 1960, a Washington newspaper carried this headline:

Silence is Ended
.... [BRADLEY] ALLOWS TEST[14]

---

[13] It is difficult to see the difference between overbearing the will of an individual through the use of so-called truth serum capable of producing incriminating evidence or a court order capable of doing the same. *Cf.,* Townsend v. Sain 372 U.S. 293 (1963); *See also generally,* J. S. MILL, ON LIBERTY, 23, (1873).

[14] A perceptive news story appeared on the same day in another Washington newspaper:

"John [Bradley] . . . accused of stabbing to death his sweetheart at [x] . . . University, has begun to cooperate with doctors trying to examine him at St. Elizabeths Hospital.

Acting Superintendent Dale C. Cameron said several staff psychiatrists and a psychologist have interviewed him in the ten days since he began talking to them . . . [Bradley], twenty, who is under indictment for first degree murder, has been examined by four doctors retained by his family. But for several months his attorney, Myron G. Ehrlich, insisted that . . . [Bradley] has a constitutional right to silence—even about his mental condition.

The government charged that [Bradley] deliberately stabbed . . . [Jane] 21, during a campus lovers' quarrel April 26. To prove guilt the government must prove that . . . [Bradley] committed the crime and had no mental disease that caused the crime.

Over defense objections last month, District Court Judge David A. Pine ordered . . . [Bradley] to cooperate with doctors who might later testify about his sanity for the prosecution. The Judge admitted, however, that he had little power to enforce such an order where an unwilling defendant is on trial for his life.

Ehrlich said he is 'positive' that 'examinations-in-depth' showed that . . . [Bradley] was of unsound mind April 26. He said . . . [Bradley] now was taking a 'calculated risk' that St. Elizabeths would agree. If the hospital disagrees, Ehrlich said, defense evidence, gathered soon after . . . [Bradley's] arrest may still prevail. Some psychiatrists are hesitant to 'date back' a diagnosis to the time several months before the examination, he noted. *(Footnote continued on next page.)*

THE DEFENDANT'S CASE TAKES SHAPE

From the start, our investigation of the case had consisted of a study of the medical reports, interviews with the defendant and his parents as well as interviews with as many of the students at the university as had first hand information about John and Jane who could be reached. Throughout May of 1960 we had spent most of our evenings interviewing students at the university. The interviews which were written up, were turned over to Dr. Salzman who, in a subsequent write-up of the case, stated that he had been greatly aided by interviews he had obtained from law students.[15]

A "guidance counselor" at the university who had been consulted by John Bradley refused all cooperation with the defense.

The following picture emerged. John's parents were well-to-do.

His father was fifty-seven and a practicing Catholic. Born in Scotland, he came to this country at the age of twenty-one to become an electrical engineer. He appeared to have no real hobby although he occasionally played golf and liked to watch television. As reported by our client, few of his father's friends ever visited them at their house.

His mother, fifty-five, was Protestant. She was a graduate nurse, and a high school teacher.

Kept almost entirely under the supervision of his mother, the boy was brought up in the Protestant faith. A slow learner, he nonetheless performed adequately in all aspects

---

. . . [Bradley's] changed conduct may avoid a showdown as to whether an accused person can refuse to give evidence about his mental condition. Assistant United States Attorney Frederick G. Smithson said he had hoped the issue would reach the United States Court of Appeals for a final ruling.

But if . . . [Bradley] is acquitted by reason of insanity, there will be no issue for appeal. Ehrlich said he would appeal Judge Pine's order if the trial results in conviction."

[15] SALZMAN, *Psychodynamics of a Case of Murder,* 3 COMPREHENSIVE PSYCHIATRY 152 (1962).

of his early schooling. His attempt at being the model boy, however, occasionally broke down. Having submitted to merciless teasing by his school mates for months at about the age of nine, he picked up an inkwell and tossed it at one of his tormentors. At eleven, he began to write long and impassioned letters to a woman school teacher, asking her to take him home with her. When she punished him for one such letter he threw her books off the desk.

He graduated from high school and then proceeded to a Junior College near his home and finally to a university in Washington, D.C.

As he put it to an examining doctor, "I always had to plug to keep up my grades so I had little time for other things." While at the university he would frequently work until 2:00 or 3:00 o'clock in the morning to maintain what he regarded as an acceptable academic average.

John met Jane at a religious club at the university. The developing relationship was a stormy one.

The interviews that we conducted with students who had known John on the university campus, confirmed the picture of an overly-conscientious boy, tormented by feelings of inadequacy, gradually approaching a breaking point under the stress of his relationship with Jane.

A fairly typical interview went as follows.

> The witness, a Miss . . . [X], had known the deceased from February of 1960 until her demise. She met John Bradley one or two nights after making the acquaintance of the deceased.
> She described . . . [Bradley] as a nice looking young man, cleancut, quiet until he got to know you, and very fond of . . . [Jane]. She then went on to say that the deceased belittled what . . . [John] was doing at every opportunity and flaunted the fact that she was going out with other boys before him as though she wanted to taunt him. The witness quoted . . . [John] as saying that he 'didn't understand why . . . [Jane] had to go out with other boys.' Still he seemed to put up with it. At first sight, as well as upon subsequent acquaintance, . . . [Bradley] proved in her view to be very sensitive and introspective.
> Miss . . . [X] recalls one particular incident in some detail. Jane was giving a party during a weekend. Bradley was one of

> the guests though Jane had also invited another young man as her date. Bradley at that time appeared almost in tears. She then corrected herself and said, It wasn't almost, he was in fact, in tears. She added that she had never observed . . . [Bradley] like that before for he always seemed in control of his emotions.
> Asked to describe . . . [Bradley] in more detail, Miss . . . [X] said that there was one element in [John] which seemed abnormal. [John] kept all emotions and feelings and frustrations to himself and let them bottle up. I didn't notice it for the most part because [John] didn't want us to notice it. Asked as to how she arrived at these conclusions, she replied: No matter what stress [John] was under, he always seemed jovial. I therefore believe that he kept all of his emotions bottled up within himself.

As events entered their climactic phase, the lights in John's room were rarely turned out before 3:00 A.M.

John consulted Miss Bess Ninaj, a religious counselor. He also sought out the university "guidance counselor" whom he asked for tranquilizers only to be told that he did not need any.

Pursuing such clues as we had concerning the events upon the campus during the last few weeks before the killing, we noted that students who had known John spoke repeatedly about an apparent increase in his agitation, starting with the month of March:

> Two boys who were jointly interviewed reported on a strange theme composed by John Bradley at that time, which they regarded as thoroughly out-of-character for him. The subject of the theme was getting out of life's rut. The defendant informed both boys that this was an independent idea of his own. On Tuesday, the day of the killing, between 11:00 and 1:00 in the afternoon he talked at great length about this new idea and his theme. At that time he seemed extremely happy and he didn't mention the girl once.
> The preceding Saturday the defendant had called the girl and had said to his friends after completing the telephone conversation: 'Boy, that really pisses me off.' The two boys remembered this remark because it was so strange an expression for the defendant to have used. He had never used that kind of language before.
> They reported that he had been getting an average number of five hours of sleep per night for at least several months.
> One boy in particular stressed that it was on Tuesday, the day of the killing, that the defendant's obsession to get out of the rut

became pronounced and unmistakable. He said he had to get off the treadmill. Although otherwise extremely tense in speech, walk and mannerism, he seemed extremely relaxed on that Tuesday. In fact, he seemed light as a dancer. I asked him about his love life and his answer was he'd take care of it.

On the Monday preceding the killing his preoccupation definitely was with his theme and not with his girl. He persisted in saying that the theme embodied his personal philosophy, his life's creed.

Our search for the essay in question bore fruit. Bradley's English instructor provided us with gratifying promptness with the following essay submitted to him on April 26, 1960, the day preceding the crime. It bore the title:

Is Life a Bore or is Man a Bore Within The Realm of Life?

It read as follows:

Today man is living in a diversified life, but because he is held to a constant and routine form of living, he sometimes is unable to touch these diversities and enjoy them. Man seems to feel that because he lives everyday the same, he has become a robot who works like an assembly line, never stopping and never going anywhere, just moving. The world moves so quickly that passing enjoyments lead only to needed wants and anxiety. When one cannot have them, he becomes bored and finally develops unhappiness.

Then again life may not be a bore, but man has made himself boring. He has not wanted to change and has considered everything to do. In *Life Magazine* last week it showed a picture in the article about the Debutante set, of a well groomed young man slouched in a chair and wearing a bored look. Here was a fellow who presumably had the social necessities, money, looks, and the fancy for women. But he was still looking for more exciting things to do. Another boy would feel that his present enjoyment was wonderful. This shows that anything can become tiresome, or that satisfaction is unattainable because some have too much and others haven't enough.

Why doesn't the human assembly line stop, let every one off and let the people do as they please until they become bored with that, and so rejuvenate with new inspirations to become a human tool of production again. Soon the diversities that were looked upon by man as enjoyment will become less exciting and new excitements will become enjoyment.

Life is a pattern which can cause people who live within

it to become stereotyped. Because of this, man has provided for such circumstances, by being creative, vacationing, and in some occasion attending movies and watching television. Not all people can become a rancher, millionaire, or beatnik. Each man must aid in the world corporation of human existence by providing for himself and looking after his interest in life. Statistically ten percent of the hundred and seventy million people in the United States are unhappy with their work. This causes boredom and mental confusion. Today man has not found himself in this fast confusing world of ours. To be born into the twentieth century means competition, hard work and enjoyment. The two previous factors are the causes for routine and continuous labor, for which the latter is a reward.

Today man can become more of a bore through his own wants rather than letting life contribute to it. Man has developed a pattern of life which we all live in. Thus man must not let himself down, and become a piece of clay which other forces can mold.

Shortly after our discovery of this essay, we secured what appeared to be an immature form of poetic prose, written by John Bradley in one of his English classes and dated April 5, 1960.

It read as follows:

GIGI

Under the spreading willow-tree, a feminine figure be. Her name is Gigi and what a beautiful girl is she. She sits with her posture very erect and a smile upon her lips. She has tender ivory skin and freckles upon her cheeks. Her hair is crisp and brown and short, her face is as white as the desert sand; She looks the whole world in the face, and tries to bring out the good in every man. Week in, week out, from morn till night, Gigi can fascinate your heart and sight. You can hear her sing in a slow, soft voice, like a birdie singing in the night. Never is there a dull moment, for she loves to play and talk. And if she does not do this, she will try to find your heart. Teasing is her feminine joy, especially to her favorite boy. For she can treat you like a toy or make you feel like you were her only joy. She always makes you feel on top, no matter if you have fallen and stopped. For she will always say, HONEST, you are the greatest. But every now and then, you must sit and explain to her, that what she has done should not have occurred. Toiling-Rejoicing-Sorrowing onward through life I go. Each morning I see her and at night also. After seeing her every day, I have earned a nights repose. Thanks,

Thanks to thee my worthy girl, for the fine times you have brought. For we will never part, and our future will be sought.

Dr. Salzman seemed enthusiastic about both discoveries but particularly the "GIGI" poem. He addressed a note to me which read as follows:

> Dick:
> This essay is fabulous. It tells the story which I have tried to piece together about his feelings, expectations, obsessional attachment, disappointment and indicates the extent of the involvement more clearly. It could almost be read *in toto* to the jury.
> Leo.

Dr. Salzman, was continuing to see the boy on a weekly basis at St. Elizabeths Hospital. He was relieved during his summer vacation by Dr. Chodoff.

As the psychoanalytic phase of the investigation by Doctors Salzman and Chodoff ground past the thirty hour mark, Dr. Chodoff telephoned me and invited me to join him at his office to discuss what he regarded as possibly a path-breaking development in the case. When I met Dr. Chodoff in his office, he appeared excited and pleased.

The investment in the intensive psychoanalytic investigation in this case, he suggested, was about to pay off. The patient, it appeared, had achieved a degree of confidence in his doctors which enabled him to produce material possibly confirmatory of active psychosis. Dr. Chodoff recounted that the patient had informed him that fellow students had called over the dormitory loudspeaker: ". . . [Bradley], Doctor Blow Job." Dr. Chodoff drew a diagram of the dormitory in which John had spent the last few months before the murder, spotting the location of the loudspeaker, and asked if I would check this out with John's neighbors so as to enable him to tell whether the experience described by John was in fact hallucinatory—as he thought it might be.

Under the impact of the self-congratulatory attitude of Dr. Chodoff I did not realize for a while that the information which he regarded as path-breaking and the payoff on some thirty hours of hard psychoanalytic work, had in fact been provided by Dr. Guttmacher as a result of a single interview.[16]

Dr. Salzman's conclusions concerning the boy combined psychiatric jargon with a style more commonly encountered in pulp fiction. The following selections seem characteristic:

> . . . In view of his background, his obsessional tendencies, his lack of self-esteem and uncertainty of his acceptability, his meeting with Jane was tragic. Tantalized by what he considered to be an attractive girl, and feeling that she had fallen for him because of her energetic pursuit of him, he fell completely for her. Finally someone liked him; in addition, he discovered that the girl was important; the daughter of an admiral. He became hopelessly and deeply committed to win her. . . .
>
> Because of the on-again, off-again nature of their relationship, he became distraught and agitated, in what could be called a dissociated state. The final straw was his inability to get her to talk to him and reassure him that all was well. Her contempt, which he read in her disgusted look, triggered a catathymic crisis and produced the irresistible impulse which led to her death.[17]

Indications were, however, that the hospital staff, to whom this was passed on, was impressed. The relations between the private psychiatrists and the staff psychiatrists, moreover, appeared good.

At our request, Dr. Salzman kept reporting on his contacts with his professional colleagues at St. Elizabeths Hospital. A typical memorandum to me as to the developing situation at St. Elizabeths read as follows:

---

[16] In his report of May 10, 1960, Dr. Guttmacher stated:
"Patient was . . . asked in what way he was kidded at . . . [the university), and he said, They called me Shrimp because of my middle name. When asked about the kidding at . . . [the] university, he said, They played all kinds of tricks on me, put water over the doorsill. They plastered all over the door and sounded out over the loudspeaker . . . [Bradley], a doctor at a blow job."

[17] Salzman, *Psychodynamics of a Case of Murder, supra* note 15.

Monday

I went to St. Elizabeths on Saturday. The situation still seems good even though I am uneasy about their having unfiled multitude of physicians reports, interviews, etc. They are being typed and will soon appear in the folder. Perhaps I can see them next Saturday. The psychologist report is very favorable to our side and I have followed your suggestion *in re* interviews with staff.

The psychologist's report states that 'under stress he has little or no control over his behavior,' and
'Break in reality could easily occur under stress.'

Will you tell Myron that it still looks good and if he wants me to talk with him directly I'll be glad to do so.

According to . . . [Bradley]; Platkin, Ward and Luik are definitely of mind that his action was 'mentally involved.' Others he's unsure about.
Could be.

Leo

I'm more and more convinced that . . . [Bradley] is an early schizophrenic of paranoid type.

FURTHER RELEVANT OR IRRELEVANT EVENTS

More than a month before the conclusion of the St. Elizabeths study, John F. Kennedy was elected President of the United States.

The local press speculated about the possible successor to Mr. Oliver Gasch, United States Attorney at the time of the Bradley indictment, and in so doing mentioned the name of Myron Ehrlich as a leading candidate for the Office.

Members of the prosecuting staff whose relations with Ehrlich and myself had been less than friendly sought us out for coffee and conversation in the courthouse cafeteria.

When I visited St. Elizabeths Hospital some time after the election I was received with greater than ordinary courtesy by Dr. Owens of the John Howard Pavilion.

In a memorandum of November 15, 1960, I reported as follows:

Owens stated that he thought . . . [Bradley] was a full-blown schizophrenic now in partial remission. He believed that he was in all likelihood in a full-blown schizophrenic state at the time of the alleged offense.

He added that he had been concerned about his earlier refusal to talk because from observing his tense reactions on the ward, he had sensed that the boy was seriously ill mentally and had felt badly about his being handicapped in his insanity defense if he did not cooperate.

Throughout the discussion Owens seemed to leave no doubt that it was his impression that the alleged crime was a product of mental illness.

THE DÉNOUEMENT AT ST. ELIZABETHS

On December 14, 1960, St. Elizabeths Hospital certified to the District Court as follows:

> . . . We conclude as a result of our examinations and observation that John S. . . . [Bradley] is mentally competent to understand the nature of the proceedings against him and to consult properly with counsel in his own defense, although he has not recovered from his mental illness. It is also our opinion that he was suffering from mental disease on or about April 26, 1960, and the criminal act, if committed by him, was probably the product of mental disease.

It was noteworthy that St. Elizabeths Hospital did not request the transfer of John Bradley to the District Jail pending the trial of his case as would have been its practice in the routine case in which such a certification was transmitted. Instead it informed us by telephone that it offered to keep the boy within its confines pending the trial and an order to that effect was entered by the District Court without opposition by the government.[18]

---

[18] One cannot help contrasting the treatment accorded to John Bradley at this time with that accorded to one John H. Strickland.

John H. Strickland was a semi-literate Negro auto mechanic, charged with the unauthorized use of a motor vehicle on or about December 15, 1960. *(Footnote continued on next page.)*

THE TRIAL

The case came to trial in January of 1961.

A jury was waived and the factual transaction charged in the indictment was stipulated.

At the time of the arrest he was an ambulatory patient at St. Elizabeths Hospital where he had spent several years.

When I saw Strickland for the first time at the District Jail he appeared in a bathrobe and told me that he had been kept in the jail hospital. He seemed completely disoriented and broke down at least twice with massive sobs. When he spoke he expressed the understanding that I was about to find some placement for him as a mechanic.

When he was brought into court, Strickland's disorientation was such as to attract the sympathetic attention of the United States Marshals. He was literally shivering with fright and had to be propelled toward the lectern fronting the judge's bench. Several times he stepped back only to be restrained.

Dr. Bernard I. Levy of the District of Columbia General Hospital, volunteered his services to interview Strickland at the jail. He informed me that he questioned Strickland's capacity to engage in rational communication with me and that he doubted the adequacy of Strickland's intellectual comprehension of his situation. He also stated that Strickland's condition appeared to have become progressively worse within the prison setting. He observed Strickland—as I had—racked by massive sobs, but also sucking his thumb throughout most of the interview.

When I contacted Dr. David Owens of the St. Elizabeths Hospital to tell him about my inability to communicate with Strickland and about Dr. Bernard Levy's impressions, Dr. Owens told me that he considered this information of no psychiatric significance.

I thereupon filed a motion for a judicial determination of Strickland's competency and for a new mental examination. The motion was supported by two affidavits: one by Dr. Bernard Levy; the other, by me. I stated that in my opinion as a lawyer, Strickland had never engaged in rational communication with me and that I therefore felt unable to render effective assistance of counsel under the circumstances.

Strickland was then recommitted to St. Elizabeths Hospital for a period of a week to ten days, with the specific request that St. Elizabeths determine his capacity to engage in rational communication with his counsel. St. Elizabeths in turn, reported back to the court that, notwithstanding the earlier certification, Strickland did not understand the indictment, the nature of the pending criminal proceedings, and that he was not capable of engaging in rational communication with his counsel.

Accordingly Strickland was adjudged not competent to stand trial
(Footnote continued on next page.)

Some evidence as to John's confession, however, was heard without objection.

Detective Sergeant Weber testified and in so doing provided a sympathetic portrayal of a youngster driven beyond his endurance.

The defense relied entirely upon the St. Elizabeths physicians to minimize further expense.

Dr. Owens testified that:

> on April 26, 1960 and even prior to that date, probably for several weeks, . . . [John] was suffering from a psychotic condition. I feel that this psychotic condition was a transitory episode, that his basic personality is one of a neurosis, psychoneurosis, obsessive-compulsive type; but that due to unusual stress, during that interval of a few weeks to a few months, around April, that date, that stress was so great that he became psychotic during that interval.

Dr. Cushard, after having stated on direct examination that in his opinion the defendant had been mentally ill on April 26, 1960 and that his crime had been a product of his mental illness, testified as follows in answer to a question by the court:

---

and was recommitted to St. Elizabeths pursuant to Section 301, Title 24, of the District of Columbia Code, in late August of 1961.

On May 25, 1962, St. Elizabeths filed a new certification stating that Strickland was competent, that he had been suffering from a psychoneurosis at the time of the alleged crime, and that no valid opinion could be propounded concerning the causal relationship between crime and illness.

When the certification came up before Chief Judge McGuire shortly after May 25, 1962, I stated to the court that I did not object to it but that I hoped an Order could be entered directing that Strickland be kept at St. Elizabeths rather than transferred to the District Jail pending the trial of his case. I informed the court that my request was prompted not only by humanitarian considerations but also by the fact that Strickland had once deteriorated to the point of incompetency to stand trial while in the jail setting. My request was denied on the ground that the court could not interfere with the internal administration of St. Elizabeths Hospital. United States v. John H. Strickland, Criminal No. 255-61 (1961).

Just a few days—I believe, if I recall correctly, it was on a Saturday, three days before the criminal act, he purchased . . . a knife, which he carried with him. He was rather vague about this. It wasn't purchased for a specific reason.

Then during the next three days, beginning on Saturday, he became so disturbed that actually he didn't know what to do, and finally he did do something which he did not want to do, but which he was afraid he would do.

Now, for some time even before this, at the university, over a period of weeks or months, he had—he spoke of some things that had been happening to him, which led me to believe that he was actually becoming psychotic. He stated that people were putting signs up regarding his alleged aberrant sexual habits, which he said were absolutely untrue; and were hanging signs out the window of McLean Gardens about the same thing, outlining the hours, as he put it, when he was open for this sort of thing; and even that one of the individuals who was one of his principal tormentors was broadcasting over a loudspeaker out the window regarding his alleged homosexual habits and activities.

Now, if these were not delusional and hallucinatory, they were so very close to it that, as I say, it is difficult to make a differentiation.

This concluded Dr. Cushard's testimony.

Dr. Mauris Platkin, the last St. Elizabeths witness to testify for the defendant, restricted himself to stating that in his opinion the defendant's act was the product of "a psychoneurotic reaction, obsessive-compulsive type."

The defense rested.

The usual motions were made.

The court thereupon proceeded to enter a judgment of acquittal by reason of insanity and to direct the hospitalization of the defendant "in accordance with the provisions of the statute."

CONCLUSION

Dr. Salzman's *whodunnit* appeared in a respected psychiatric periodical.

As he saw it, the end result was entirely attributable to the "cooperative endeavor" between the psychiatrists for the defense and those of St. Elizabeths Hospital and the consequent avoidance of the "usual contentious situation."[19] In this light the role of the lawyers might almost be viewed as irrelevant to, if not actually obstructive of, the happy outcome.

I, of course, see the matter very differently.

But the reader is perhaps best left to draw his own conclusions.

---

[19] Salzman, *Psychodynamics of a Case of Murder, supra* note 15.

Chapter VI

THE DEFENSE OF WALTER X. WILSON: AN INSANITY PLEA AND A SKIRMISH IN THE WAR ON POVERTY

It is commonplace to observe that with the best lawyer in the world a man may lose a case that he ought to win for lack of a happy pairing of merit and money.

In a criminal case, lack of money may mean not only loss of liberty but actual loss of life. Whether or not Walter X. Wilson[1] had a good lawyer is in this light less important than whether or not he had adequate financial resources to assert his innocence. What emerges with startling clarity is that, but for the bounty of the National Institute of Mental Health, Walter X. Wilson would have gone to a penitentiary instead of a mental hospital.

Walter X. Wilson's story is told in part as an illustration of the adage that regardless of applicable legal doctrine—and the *M'Naghten* rule would no more have affected the outcome of this case than the *Durham* rule—"money talks." It is also told with a view to presenting a clearer identification of the problems faced by counsel in the preparation of the insanity defense, for again—regardless of the prevailing rule of exculpatory mental illness in a particular jurisdiction—counsel will generally face substantially identical attitudes within the hierarchy of the state mental institution and experience much the same type of pitfalls in com-

---

[1] A pseudonym has been substituted for the name of the defendant, therefore no attempt is made to support any colloquies by reference to the actual transcripts.

munication with the experts of his own selection which were encountered in the Wilson case.

MANSLAUGHTER UPON THE HIGHWAY

At about 3:00 A.M. on Thursday, June 9, 1960, Precinct No. 8 of the Washington, D.C. Police Department was informed that a stolen car had been seen passing through a red light on Missouri Avenue.

A police patrol car was alerted and pursued a Chevrolet station wagon which had been identified as the stolen car. As the police car pulled abreast of the station wagon, a police officer motioned it over to the curb. The station wagon, driven by nineteen year-old Walter X. Wilson, sped away.

The police officer sounded his siren and the chase began. Walter X. Wilson was driving his car at an estimated speed of eighty miles per hour and was weaving from side to side on the street.

The blocking of the roadway by a police car in advance of Wilson's careening vehicle as an alternative to pursuit was thought by an officer of the Accident Investigation Unit as "taking . . . his own life in . . . [his] hands and maybe anybody else's life who was with . . . [him]."

The pursuit covered approximately three miles over a winding road, moving uphill and then down again.

In the 3700 block of Military Road, Walter X. Wilson's station wagon collided head-on with a Chevrolet sedan coming from the opposite direction, driving the sedan back seventy-four feet into a third car. In the process, Wilson's station wagon turned over in the air "and continued eighty-four feet, ending up-right against a tree with [its] tailgate . . . against the tree and the front end protruding . . . in a westerly direction on Military Road."

All four occupants of the Chevrolet sedan were killed.

Three were dead on arrival at a local hospital; one died within minutes of his hospitalization.

Walter X. Wilson was brought, unconscious and in critical condition, to the George Washington University Hospital for emergency treatment. His injuries included cerebral concussion, multiple lacerations and multiple fractures. After passing the critical stage, he was transferred to the D.C. General Hospital for further treatment.

His physical condition did not permit him to participate in the Coroner's inquest until October 5, 1960. The Coroner's jury found him responsible for the death of the four occupants of the sedan and ordered him held for action of the Grand Jury. The Grand Jury indicted him on four counts of manslaughter, which in the words of the indictment, was attributable to his driving a station wagon "feloniously, wantonly and with gross negligence . . ."

Subsequent to his indictment, he was transferred to the prison hospital of the District of Columbia jail.

The first lawyer appointed to represent him received leave to withdraw from the case. Apparently the boy had refused to cooperate. The same thing happened in the case of the second appointed lawyer. I was the third appointed.

Walter was brought from the jail hospital into the rotunda to be interviewed by his new counsel. He was painfully limping about on his crutches and seated himself with some difficulty at the table reserved for conferences with counsel. I introduced myself, and after some inconsequential preliminary discussion, asked my client if he would like to tell me about the accident. Wilson's monosyllabic response was *"No."*

I did not press him to engage in a discussion which he was clearly bent upon avoiding and proceeded instead to inquire about his physical condition and the way in which he was being treated by the jail authorities. He relaxed slightly in response to these questions and provided some inconsequential information.

About this time, I received a telephone call from my

counterpart in the United States Attorney's office informing me that the prosecution would move for a mental examination of the boy on the ground that he had been previously hospitalized as a psychiatric patient, and inquiring if the defense would object. I replied that I would join in the motion of the government.

Neither defense nor prosecuting counsel knew, at this stage, that while the boy had indeed been a psychiatric patient at the D.C. General and St. Elizabeths Hospital in 1956, a sharp split of opinion had existed between the two hospitals at that time. The D.C. General Hospital had certified the patient as psychotic and in need of hospitalization; St. Elizabeths Hospital had certified him as free from mental disorder and had recommended his discharge.

The present commitment for mental observation was to St. Elizabeths Hospital.

THUMBNAIL SKETCH OF A "KILLER"

The defense investigation of this case consisted of a study of all available court and hospital records, interviews with friends, relatives and employers, further interviews with the boy, independent psychiatric examinations, as well as psychiatric examinations on court order at the D.C. General Hospital after the conclusion of the St. Elizabeths examination.

In aid of this investigation I moved for, and obtained a court order directing St. Elizabeths Hospital and the D.C. General Hospital to furnish me with photostatic copies of all records of Walter Wilson at the expense of the United States.

Photostatic copies of the D.C. General Hospital records of Walter's hospitalization in 1956 were promptly and courteously forwarded to me. St. Elizabeths Hospital did not follow suit.

A few days passed. I was having coffee in the courthouse cafeteria and was joined at my table by the Assistant U.S. Attorney in charge of the prosecution. As we chatted, the prosecutor told me with a smile that he had just been contacted by Dr. Overholser, the Superintendent of St. Elizabeths, and told that he should have *resisted* my request for the hospital records. Dr. Overholser had gone on to explain to the prosecuting counsel that he greatly feared that I would use the hospital records to "upset" the "patient." I replied that Dr. Overholser was more likely to fear that I would use the hospital records to upset the hospital staff. We then went on to discuss Washington's entertainment scene.

The boy's history, as gleaned from a lawyer's investigation, can be summarized as follows:

The boy's parents were married in their teens. His father, who himself had had numerous brushes with the law, including a conviction for impersonating a federal officer, was an alcoholic. His mother had held down menial jobs throughout most of her life. She apparently received no financial support from her husband. When Walter was eight years old his mother, at that time expecting her fourth child, left her husband and went to live with her mother. It was clear (even upon cursory interviewing), that she was a person of low average intelligence with extreme hostility toward the boy. As I left her at the conclusion of an interview, she declared:

> And be sure to tell me when the trial is to be held because I want to be there to see Walter convicted.

During the first year of Walter's life his mother became the breadwinner of the family while the father remained at home to mind the baby. Apparently, he minded the bottle rather than the baby, with the result that the child was discovered dirty and unfed upon the mother's return at night. During the first year of Walter's life he began hitting his head against the wall for hours on end. He would usually not stop, even though his head was bleeding. He had also developed dietary difficulties. One was his refusal to swallow food. During the next few years he began "rocking and rolling himself to sleep" in a rhythmic fashion which he subsequently exhibited with dramatic results in the courtroom before a startled judge and jury. His mother reported that he had intense sleeping difficulties beginning with the first years of his life and that by the time he had reached adolescence he was rarely able to sleep more than four hours a night. Early in his childhood he was witness to violent quarrels between his parents.

His difficulties with authority figures, already pronounced at home, manifested themselves in his school environment. He was sent to a Catholic parochial school, from which he was expelled for breaking into a church poorbox. He said that all of his subsequent troubles were attributable to the harsh discipline imposed upon him by the Sisters.

His experience with the public school system was no more satisfactory. He would arrive at school dirty, unkempt and fatigued from apparent lack of sleep. He did poorly in his studies, drawing being the only subject which appeared to interest him.

It was his view that he was the object of some sort of conspiracy at that time. Early in his school days he developed an acute fear of the police officers of Precinct No. 8 who, he believed, were plotting to "nail him to the door." He was involved in various acts of delinquency and spent some time at the National Training School for Boys.

At the age of fifteen he approached a girl in school with a knife. He later explained that he had to get her before she got him. The Juvenile Court sent him to the D.C. General Hospital for psychiatric observation. This hospital kept him for four months and a diagnostic staff conference concluded that he was psychotic, needing hospitalization. A certification to this effect was transmitted to the Juvenile Court, which accepted it and committed the boy to St. Elizabeths Hospital where he was kept for a little over three weeks. The hospital records covering that period show little diagnostic contact beyond some psychological testing. Although the results of the psychological testing were reported in the hospital records as indicating a very precariously balanced individual, "desperately" in need of psychotherapy, the hospital reported him to be suffering from nothing more serious than a minor adolescent disturbance and discharged him.

Several years before the automobile collision he had been expelled from his home by his mother and had since led a hand-to-mouth existence, shifting from job to job, and frequently living in alleyways, garages and public parks.

Neighbors furnished the information that he had developed a bizarre liking for dog food. When offered a sandwich by a neighbor, he would refuse it but would steal dog food when he thought the neighbor was not looking. His last reported job was in a veterinary hospital, where he became addicted to dog tranquilizers. He also drank heavily. While at the veterinary hospital, he expressed the fear that he was under constant surveillance by the police and complained about being shadowed by a police spy, whom he identified. The "spy" turned out to be an innocuous, retired old man who was in the habit of sunning himself outside the veterinary hospital.

The immediate events preceding the accident are not wholly clear but this much can be claimed with some degree of reliability:

There was an increase in the intake of alcohol and dog tranquilizers.

The boy made some attempt to join the Army, but was told that he was not eligible because of his police record.

He looked more than usually depressed.

On the day of the accident he was accosted in a bar by a homosexual. He had just taken five dog tranquilizers and had had approximately nine glasses of beer to wash them down. It was not clear as to precisely what transpired between him and the homosexual beyond the fact that he felt that some homosexual overture had been made to him. It was clear that he had entered the homosexual's car, that a tussle ensued and that the homosexual was thrown out. Walter then proceeded to drive the car away for the purpose, as he put it, of "splattering myself all over the sidewalk so the police would have a mess to clean up."

The coroner's transcript revealed that the police had been notified of a stolen car and had pulled abreast of one matching its description. The car, driven by Walter X. Wilson had until that time been proceeding at normal speed. When the police car pulled abreast of him, Walter cast one look in its direction and stepped upon his accelerator. As previously noted, the car reached the speed of eighty miles per hour and weaved erratically from lane to lane until it collided with one approaching from the opposite direction, killing four people and inflicting nearly fatal injuries upon Walter himself.

While hospitalized for his injuries Walter collected approximately ten sleeping pills. He consumed all of these on one night. His stomach was pumped and the notation included in his record by an intern that he seemed to require psychiatric supervision. Shortly before this abortive suicidal attempt, he had informed a nurse that he had a knife and was going to "get her" with it. The nurse summoned the intern on duty to conduct a search of the room, but no knife was found.

A DEFENSE TAKES SHAPE

I secured the services of Dr. Leon Salzman, of the Washington School of Psychiatry, and Dr. Edward Sachar, a psychiatrist on the staff of the Walter Reed Hospital.

Dr. Sachar interviewed the boy for several hours while he was still at the District jail, and diagnosed him as an aggressive and impulsive psychopath. While he was prepared to state that he regarded Walter's action as the product of a mental illness, he described his patient in such uncomplimentary language that I preferred to forego his testimony.

Dr. Salzman interviewed the patient more briefly at St. Elizabeths Hospital and stated without hesitation that he diagnosed him as suffering from schizophrenia, paranoid type.

In my contacts with Dr. Salzman I indicated my particular interest in a psychoanalytically-oriented development of the study of Walter X. Wilson, which would be acceptable to a lay jury. At the doctor's request, I furnished him with an excerpt from the *Carter* case, to the specific effect that:

> the chief value of an expert's testimony in this field . . . rests upon the material from which his opinion is fashioned . . . ; in the explanation of the disease and its dynamics, that is, how it arose, developed and affected the mental and emotional process of the defendant.[2]

Dr. Salzman was not unfamiliar with this approach. He had in fact furnished an affidavit in an earlier case stating that a particular series of examinations undertaken by him was "designed to provide a view in depth of the defendant's mental and emotional processes" and expressing his "professional opinion that such examinations in depth . . . [could] be adequately conducted only by intensive psychoanalytic techniques."

Prior to the trial he examined the defendant on two further occasions.

I also contacted Dr. John D. Schultz, the Medical Director of the D.C. General Hospital, who had conducted the initial psychiatric examination of 1956. Dr. Schultz stated that it was highly unlikely that the boy's mental condition would have cleared up without treatment, and, upon hearing the description of the events leading to the boy's arrest, declared it probable that the boy's illness had taken a turn for the worse. He offered to cooperate with any doctors in charge of the mental examination.

---

[2] Carter v. United States, 252 F.2d 608, 617 (D.C. Cir. 1957).

Acting without objection from the United States Attorney's office, I moved for a court order directing Dr. John D. Schultz to examine Walter Wilson with a view to updating his initial findings.

Thereafter I informed several of the St. Elizabeths physicians examining my client that I had a fairly elaborate social history on the boy which I would submit to them upon request. I further informed them that Doctors Salzman and Schultz would confer with them in aid of their diagnostic evaluation.

Finally, toward the end of Walter's three month period of hospitalization at St. Elizabeths, I requested the complete record of Walter's hospitalization in 1956 and also the new hospital record upon its completion. Up to this time, there had been no response from St. Elizabeths to my request for data on any level whatsoever.

When the three month period of hospitalization at St. Elizabeths had approximately a week to run, and there still had been no compliance by St. Elizabeths with the court order directing the transmission of the hospital records to the defense, I wrote directly to the Superintendent of St. Elizabeths Hospital renewing the request for complete hospital records and stressing the urgency of the situation.

More or less five days before the trial date, Dr. Mauris Platkin of St. Elizabeths telephoned and informed me that the hospital had found Walter Wilson to be without mental disorder, and that copies of the hospital records would be sent to me "in due course." We were disconnected almost immediately and I was unable to reach Dr. Platkin for several hours. When I did, I urged again the importance of my receiving the records immediately so that my experts would have an opportunity for study and independent evaluation a few days before trial. Dr. Platkin refused. He declared that nothing could be done to speed up normal hospital procedures. I responded by saying that I would be constrained to bring contempt proceedings if the records were not delivered within the next two days.

Within two days the records were delivered to me by special government messenger.

When finally received, the photostatic copies were incomplete. The results of psychological testing were missing. I called St. Elizabeths to inquire about the missing report and was told that no psychological tests had been run. When I asked to speak to the Chief of Service, Dr. Cushard, I was told that Dr. Cushard was suffering from laryngitis and that he could not speak to me. I retorted again that I would be constrained to bring contempt proceedings. Two hours later I received a photostatic copy of the psychological report.[3]

The psychological report concluded that Walter Wilson was a schizophrenic. The balance of the hospital record showed two psychiatric interviews of undetermined duration, notwithstanding the certification to the court that the defendant had been studied intensively since his admission date.

Shortly thereafter St. Elizabeths Hospital transmitted its official certification to the court that Walter Wilson was without mental disorder. The relevant portion of the St. Elizabeths certification read as follows:

> . . . Mr. [Wilson's] case has been studied intensively since the date of his admission to Saint Elizabeths Hospital and he has been examined by several qualified psychiatrists attached to the medical staff of Saint Elizabeths Hospital as to his mental condition. On February 15, 1961, Mr. [Walter X. Wilson] was examined and the case reviewed in detail at a medical staff

---

[3] The difficulties encountered in securing medical records to which defense counsel was legally entitled were in no way unique. Dr. Morton Birnbaum, testifying before the Senate Subcommittee on Constitutional Rights, related a comparable experience which he encountered in seeking the release (through a *habeas corpus* proceeding) of his indigent client from Creedmore Hospital in New York State. Dr. Birnbaum requested the hospital records of his client in July, 1960. After three months of delay by the hospital and the lawyer from the Attorney General's office, he was finally allowed to inspect his client's hospital records. *Hearings before the Subcommittee on Constitutional Rights of the Committee of the Judiciary,* United States Senate, 87th Cong., 1st Sess., at 298, 299 (1961).

conference. We conclude, as a result of our examination and observation, that Mr. [Walter X. Wilson] is mentally competent to understand the nature of the proceedings against him and consult properly with counsel in his own defense. We find no evidence of mental disease existing at the present time nor on or about June 8, 1960. He is not suffering from mental deficiency.

On February 16, 1961, a day after that certification and after the defendant had been removed to the D.C. jail and the trial "continued," Dr. Platkin contacted Dr. Salzman. The latter's memorandum to me on his conversation with Dr. Platkin reads as follows:

> 4:30 P.M. Dr. Platkin called to ask if I had seen Mr. [Wilson] and whether I had some data that might be useful to them. . . . Since they already held their staff conference I suggested that the data could not serve the same purpose as if it were given before the conference. He said they would change their minds if new data were supplied. . . .

I asked Dr. Salzman directly whether he thought that Dr. Platkin and the others at St. Elizabeths had an open mind or whether they were merely trying to fortify their conclusion that there was no mental disorder by saying that they had taken every relevant medical view into account. Dr. Salzman replied that he did not think the St. Elizabeths people had an open mind on the case. I instructed him therefore not to transmit any information to them.

It was clear at this stage that St. Elizabeths Hospital would furnish articulate and court-experienced psychiatrists to testify that the defendant was without mental disorder. The impact of such testimony would be overwhelming in the absence of flagrant and overtly detectable symptoms of psychotic psychopathology, particularly in view of the claim which would be made that the St. Elizabeths opinion was based upon intensive studies carried out during ninety days of observation and examination in a hospital setting immediately preceding the trial—a claim which would clearly not be matched by the available defense psychiatrists.

One means of balancing the scales more favorably in the interest of the defendant appeared to be to have him re-examined by the staff of the D.C. General Hospital's Psychiatric Division. But as a practical matter, a presumption of regularity attached to the completion of a mental examination at St. Elizabeths Hospital and barring a showing of extraordinary cause, I could not hope for re-examination in a new hospital setting.

However, I had available to me the opinion of Dr. Schultz that a hospital setting was needed to complete the examination of the defendant to his own professional satisfaction. The photostatic copies of the records forwarded from St. Elizabeths Hospital showed the absence of an electroencephalogram. Sympathy for brain damage—if not for psychological harm—seemed widespread within the District Court. Failure to check upon the possible existence of brain damage as a consequence of the concussion suffered by the defendant struck me as persuasive support for a new mental examination.

In an unopposed motion for Walter's commitment to the D.C. General Hospital Psychiatric Division, I reiterated Dr. Schultz's assertion concerning his inability to do an adequate study without further hospitalization and pointed to the failure of St. Elizabeths Hospital to administer an electroencephalogram in a case of cerebral concussion.

On February 27, 1961, The District Court directed the transfer of the defendant to the D.C. General Hospital Psychiatric Division for a period of four days. As a consequence of that transfer, the defendant gained the additional support of the following prospective witnesses: Dr. John D. Schultz, formerly the Chief Psychiatrist and at the time of the trial Medical Director of the D.C. General Hospital, who in 1956 had diagnosed the boy as psychotic and who now brought his findings up to date, and Dr. Bernard Levy, the Chief Psychologist of the D.C. General Hospital. Both regarded the boy as psychotic and his "crime" a product of his disorder.

I had hoped that the transfer of the accused to the D.C. General Hospital would result in recruitment of more than these two witnesses. However, under the court order the commitment was for only four days and the Chief Psychiatrist of the D.C. General Hospital stated that she could not make any further staff members available for the case in that brief time span. It was clear at this stage that my main concern was not solely that of gathering further testimonial support, but rather that of obtaining a solid institutional front of D.C. General psychiatrists for this case. Opposed by one government hospital, it seemed vital to obtain another government hospital completely committed to the insanity defense. Available National Institute of Mental Health funds were utilized to retain Dr. James A. Ryan, Assistant Chief Psychiatrist at D.C. General Hospital, with this end in view. His "recruitment" did not take place until the boy's transfer from the D.C. General Hospital to the District of Columbia jail. Dr. Ryan, of course, utilized the available D.C. General Hospital records in aid of his diagnostic evaluation since his diagnostic contacts with the boy were restricted to examinations conducted at the jail before and during the trial.[4] Another staff member of the D.C. General Hospital "recruited" for the case was a psychologist

---

[4] "In general, the observation of a criminal made during the fatal hours preceding the trial, reveals to a psychoanalyst a great deal about the unconscious of the man; at times even more is revealed than in the course of many empty weeks of a difficult analysis of a psychoneurotic. The dramatically concentrated expressions of the man's unconscious, just before and during the trial, are more convincing at times and much deeper than the protracted epic presentation which the unconscious uses in free association."

F. ALEXANDER & H. STAUB, THE CRIMINAL, THE JUDGE AND THE PUBLIC 137 (1956).

As a layman I cannot, of course, make any valid generalizations concerning the significance of Dr. Ryan's *locus* of examination in this case beyond setting forth the view quoted above. But I *can* state that apparently more experienced psychiatrists with identical opportunities for observation in the prison failed to match the intuitive and intellectual understanding displayed by Dr. Ryan in this case.

who had initially tested the boy in 1956. Both concluded that the boy was schizophrenic and that his psychopathology had triggered the act charged in the indictment.

At about this time, two dissenters within the framework of the St. Elizabeths hierarchy indicated willingness to testify for the defense. They were Dr. Brigitte Julian, who believed the boy to be mentally ill but felt that she had not had an opportunity to make a more precise diagnosis; and Dr. Catherine Beardsley, the Chief of Training in Psychology at St. Elizabeths, who believed the boy to be schizophrenic.

I further attempted to secure a psychiatrist who would be willing, perhaps even without examining the defendant, to give the court his own evaluation of the adequacy of the diagnostic work-up at St. Elizabeths Hospital, as reflected by its records. Approximately six reputable psychiatrists in the District of Columbia were approached on this subject but all refused to consider it. One well-known local psychiatrist expressed outright shock and amazement at the mere *thought* that a lawyer would consider a maneuver by which a psychiatric witness could be called upon to criticize the adequacy of the diagnostic work-up at St. Elizabeths Hospital.

Out-of-town psychiatrists had to be contacted. One agreed to do an evaluation of this kind. Unexpectedly, however, we secured the services of Dr. Charles Goshen, at that time an Assistant Professor of Psychiatry at George Washington University Medical School and a former administrator in the hierarchy of the American Psychiatric Association. Dr. Goshen agreed to review the St. Elizabeths Hospital records but insisted upon examining the defendant himself. His conclusion was that the accused was clearly schizophrenic and that the records reflected an inadequate diagnostic work-up, although such data as were available to St. Elizabeths pointed to the presence of a schizophrenic illness.

A word or two about the defense counsel's contacts with the defense experts in advance of trial is in order at this point.

I discussed the case with Dr. Schultz in an interview that lasted approximately fifteen minutes. He stated without any ambiguity that he regarded the patient as schizophrenic and suggested that the failure of St. Elizabeths Hospital to recognize the schizophrenic process might be attributable to an excessive preoccupation with a quest for *secondary* as distinct from *primary* symptoms of schizophrenia. Since Walter Wilson often did not seem to manifest such secondary symptoms as hallucinatory experiences, it was possible that *hurried* examination or examination by *inadequately* trained or *inexperienced* psychiatrists might fail to turn up the proper diagnostic data. He observed, in the wry tone of a lecturer, that psychiatrists no longer required a finding of secondary symptoms for a diagnosis of schizophrenia and that the diagnosis of schizophrenia upon the basis of primary symptoms was a subject of frequent questioning on examinations conducted by the American Board of Psychiatry and Neurology.[5]

I saw Dr. Salzman about this case briefly on approximately three occasions. In addition, he furnished me with three written reports on his examinations. He initially described his patient as:

> . . . a rather tight-lipped, unfriendly and anxious person, who cooperated in the interview but used the occasion largely to defend and justify his situation.[6]

---

[5] Bleuler's classic treatment of the schizophrenic process provides the following information in this field:

"We can only understand a psychically determined psychosis if we distinguish the symptoms stemming directly from the disease process itself from those secondary symptoms which only begin to operate when the sick psyche reacts to some internal or external processes."

E. BLEULER, DEMENTIA PRAECOX OR THE GROUP SCHIZOPHRENIAS 348 (1950).

[6] Salzman, *Psychiatric Interviews as Evidence: The Role of the Psychiatrist in Court—Some Suggestions and Case Histories*, 30 GEO. WASH. L. REV. 853, 862-864 (1962).

Dr. Salzman's findings were highlighted in these words:

"There is a clear atmosphere of intense hostility radiating to everyone, but particularly the police. This is strong enough and embracing enough to justify being called a paranoid system. He insists that the three detectives
(Footnote continued on next page.)

Dr. Salzman did, at my request, confer with two of the lay witnesses who had known the defendant. He showed no interest in the defendant's intake of dog tranquilizers and nine glasses of beer. I suggested to Dr. Salzman that he describe the boy to the jury as though he were talking about him to a group of mildly interested but unsophisticated relatives concerned about how they could help.

Dr. Ryan conferred with me at great length, both in personal conferences and over the telephone. He took the initiative in contacting people who had known the boy and telephoned the Edgemoor Animal Hospital to determine the content of the tranquilizers he had taken. Prior to his testimony in the courtroom, Dr. Ryan asked to see his patient within the cell block. He readily conferred with me in the courtroom corridor about the boy's problems and his views of the case. He appeared to be the only physician, in addition to Dr. Charles Goshen, to manifest a concern over the boy's ability to cope with the continuing stress of the trial.

In preparing to meet the psychiatric evidence of the

---

from No. 8 Precinct had it in for him and hated him and threatened frequently to kill him. While he could not explain why they hated him, and he recognized that he was in much trouble before meeting them, he insists that they are responsible for all his trouble, since they provoked and tormented him. There appears to be no hallucination at the time, but there is a rather elaborate delusional system, with the accompanying intense hatred that could easily be fanned into homicide.

His attitude is arrogant and contemptuous and while he appears to have no remorse for the fatal accident, he is tense and anxious to a point of exaggerated control which periodically breaks down, when he becomes angry, threatening and insulting."

A subsequent report by Dr. Salzman provided little historical explanation of the defendant's mental state but confirmed the impression of psychotic psychopathology.

Thus the patient was described as follows on March 5, 1961:

"On this occasion he was sullen, flattened in affect and quite withdrawn. He said No. 8 Precinct was planning to shoot him and nail him to a door. He has had no rest from the police and if he had the opportunity he would kill them all. He says he has also killed lots of people mentally. He trusts nobody. The paranoid ideas are more firmly clarified on this occasion, with some suggestion of hallucination regarding his father. He again expresses his excessive fury at homosexuality."

prosecution, which would, of course, conform with St. Elizabeths Hospital's findings of "no mental disorder," the defense planned to emphasize what we considered to be the failings of St. Elizabeths psychiatric workup; first, a lack of a psychiatric examination in depth, as well as a lack of a psychoanalytically trained psychiatrist to conduct such an examination (Dr. Salzman was expected to testify as to the requirements of an examination in depth which would provide more than a descriptive label); second, the refusal of St. Elizabeths to avail itself of the substantial data concerning the defendant's life history gathered by the defense investigation.

THE FIRST DAY OF THE TRIAL

I had decided upon the following seating arrangement. I seated myself at the head of the counsel table. Two law students assisting me in the case were seated to my right. The defendant, Walter X. Wilson, was the next man on the right. Sitting behind him was the marshal who was assigned to guard him. Flanking Walter upon the extreme right hand corner was my associate counsel.

The decision as to seating was prompted by the feeling that any closer proximity between counsel and client would result in needlessly distracting pleas for information from the latter. I also felt that conferences between counsel and client at counsel table were regarded by the average jury as evidence of rational participation inconsistent with an insanity defense.[7] Accordingly, I instructed my associate and his two student assistants not to initiate any conversation with Walter but to jot down any request that he might make during the trial and pass it on to me.

The opening note, struck by the introductory remarks of

---

[7] *See e.g.*, United States v. Stewart, Crim. No. 633-53 (D.D.C. 1962) Transcript of Proceedings, at 2204.

prosecuting counsel to the prospective jury members, was casual and relaxed.

Walter, who had initially been fixing his eyes on the floor, subsequently allowed himself to slump over the counsel table, burying his head in his arms. A marshal approached me at that stage and whispered that the judge wanted the defendant to sit up. I so instructed Walter. Walter followed directions but later lapsed into his earlier position. Thereafter his position at the counsel table could be best described in the words of a visiting psychologist:

> While sitting in his straight chair, the defendant rocked rhythmically back and forth, his entire trunk and head moving to and fro in a steady, mechanical motion.[8]

I inquired on *voir dire* whether the prospective jurors might be "adversely affected against the defendant in the evaluation of an insanity defense if there should be evidence, as well there might be, that the defendant . . . [had] been involved in acts of juvenile delinquency as a child."

The court interrupted to inquire how I intended to bring that out. I replied that some of the psychiatrists would base their final diagnostic opinion in part upon a history of protracted maladjustment, including juvenile delinquency and that this delinquency would be considered only as one of a large number of symptoms all of which, viewed in their totality, impelled a given doctor to a particular conclusion.

I inquired at another point whether the prospective jurors would be prepared to return a verdict of not guilty by reason of insanity even if the defendant did not resemble a wild beast.

There was silence.

I responded that I gathered that they would indeed "be prepared to acquit on the basis of a reasonable doubt as to mental illness and its connection with the crime, even

---

[8] Scheflen, *The Psychologist as a Witness,* 32 PENN. BAR Ass'N Q. 329 (1961).

though the defendant . . . [was] not shown to be a wild beast or bereft of reason in any way."

The jury as finally composed consisted of a program analyst, an unemployed clerk typist, a "contact representative," three housewives, a male room attendant, a "press man," an analyst, a scientific instructor, an economist and a retired gentleman. Negroes and whites were represented about equally on the jury.

The factual transaction was promptly stipulated by the defense and prosecution in open court:

THE PROSECUTION: It is stipulated between counsel that in the early morning hours of June 9, 1960, I believe at about 2:40 A.M., the evidence will establish that one Julian Thompson was driving his automobile in an easterly direction in the 3700 block of Military Road, Northwest, in the District of Columbia;

That . . . in the front seat of the automobile was one Constantine Poulos; in the rear left side behind the driver was one John W. Morris;

In the middle, in the back, was Charles Williams;

And on the right side was Edward F. Johaneck.

The evidence will establish that when they had arrived at that point and traveling in an orderly manner and within the speed limit, . . . there was an oncoming car which had been observed at Missouri Avenue in the District of Columbia going in a westerly direction;

That this automobile began picking up speed when it had come under the observation of members of the Police Department in a squad car.

The evidence will establish that it proceeded along Military Road, Northwest, going in a westerly direction; that it had weaved to the right and to the left; that it had arrived at speeds in excess of sixty miles an hour.

The evidence will establish, or it is stipulated, that when it arrived, these cars came together at 2701 Military Road, Northwest, in the District of Columbia, there was a head-on collision.

The point of impact in this collision would show that the automobile going in a westerly direction was a couple feet south of the center line which would put it in line of the oncoming car that was going in the easterly direction in which the aforementioned deceased mentioned in the indictments were traveling.

The point of impact would also show that the car going in the easterly direction in which the deceased was, was slightly over the center line.

The evidence further stipulated—

THE COURT: Which car was over the center line?
THE PROSECUTION: Both of them.
THE COURT: Both of them were over the center line?
THE PROSECUTION: Yes, sir.
THE COURT: Very well.
THE PROSECUTION: The evidence further showed that from the point of impact the automobile in which the four deceased were, along with this John W. Norris, was forced back approximately seventy-eight feet.

The evidence would show that at the time of the collision that this automobile being driven by the defendant [Walter X. Wilson] going at a highly excessive rate of speed and that just prior to the collision it had weaved to the right and to the left excessively.

The evidence will further be, or is, that the officers on arriving at the scene did see the defendant in the striking vehicle which had been going in the westerly direction;

That he was taken from that automobile and taken to the hospital for treatment.

The facts are and the evidence is that . . . [the four occupants of the other vehicle were all pronounced dead on arrival at nearby hospitals within one hour of the collision].

The evidence will show further to the effect that . . . the next morning Dr. Welton, Deputy Coroner in and for the District of Columbia, made an autopsy of the remains of the four deceased described in the indictment, and which I have already told you were taken from the automobile;

That this autopsy was that the injuries that these aforementioned sustained did cause their death and that these injuries were sustained in this automobile accident on the morning of June 9, 1960.

Following a conference at the bench, it was further stipulated that the defendant had begun to speed and weave from one lane to another only after a police car had approached him and that this approach was justified in view of the stolen car report. In addition, the injuries sustained by the defendant, as indicated by certain hospital records, were agreed upon.

In my opening statement to the jury, I observed:

> There were warning signs . . . of mental illness [in the case of Walter X. Wilson]. These warning signs were ignored. . . .
> In 1956, the boy, after numerous episodes of bizarre, acute, and dramatic maladjustment, was sent to the D.C. General Hospital Psychiatric Division, where he spent four months and received the intensive . . . attention of the doctors, headed by Dr. John D. Schultz, who will testify before you.
> And it was at that time, in 1956, when the boy was only fifteen . . . that Dr. Schultz reported . . . that the boy was . . . psychotic . . . and that society's interest demanded that he be confined in a hospital where treatment was available, and where he could be cured of his illness. . . .
> Dr. Schultz's warning fell on deaf ears.
> The boy was released from St. Elizabeths. . . .

My first two witnesses were Dr. Schultz and Dr. Salzman. Both had nervously paced the corridor adjoining the courtroom while awaiting their call. Both expressed displeasure at their loss of time.

Dr. Schultz was the first witness for the defense and was called immediately following a recess.[9] His testimony was couched essentially in conclusory terms and depended for its persuasiveness essentially upon his authoritative and self-assured air and presentation.

Dr. Schultz observed that he had diagnosed the defendant as schizophrenic in 1956 and that his present opinion was substantially the same. It was his further opinion that the defendant's crimes, if any, were the products of his mental illness.

Dr. Schultz had difficulty recalling aspects of the case at certain times and struggled with his recollection of details. This deficiency became particularly apparent upon redirect examination. The following is illustrative.

THE DEFENSE: Aside from the diagnosis of any other doctor, Dr. Schultz, is there anything within the hospital record during the period indicated, June to September, 1960, suggestive of mental disturbance? And I refer to what the defendant is reported to have done, rather than anything that may have been said about his condition on psychiatric study.

THE WITNESS: I can't answer that. I would have to restudy it. I don't recall that there is and I don't recall that there is not.

THE DEFENSE: Dr. Schultz, is it not a fact that the hospital record between June and September, 1960, reflects an

---

[9] Once the stipulation had been made in open court, the government's case as to the facts of the manslaughter charge was established. It then became incumbent on the defense to introduce "some evidence" of mental disorder in the accused, which the government in turn had to disprove beyond a reasonable doubt if it were to secure a guilty verdict. Tatum v. United States, 190 F.2d 612 615 (D.C. Cir. 1951). This explains the topsy-turvy sequence of witnesses in this case, with the defense calling the first witness and the prosecution following with its evidence as to the accused's sanity.

attempted suicide by the defendant [Walter X. Wilson]?
THE WITNESS: There is a note to that effect in the record; that is correct.
THE PROSECUTION: Does that have some significance for you, Doctor?
THE WITNESS: No, sir.
THE DEFENSE: Dr. Schultz, you do not consider suicidal attempts to be evidence of mental health, do you sir?
THE PROSECUTION: I object to that—this suicidal attempt, in this case.
THE DEFENSE: Very well, in this case.
THE WITNESS: Evidence of emotional disturbance, yes, but this can occur in any diagnostic setting. That is why I said it had no special diagnostic significance.

Upon the resumption of the trial that afternoon following a luncheon recess, Dr. Salzman took the stand. I established his qualifications, including a teaching position at St. Elizabeths Hospital which allowed him to assert that the staff members of the John Howard Pavilion were generally present or former students of his "because they come through ... [his] seminar."

A lack of rapport between Dr. Salzman and myself appeared evident almost immediately:

THE DEFENSE: Do you have an opinion, Dr. Salzman, to a reasonable medical certainty, as to whether the accident described in the indictment, ... was a product of the mental illness which you have diagnosed?
THE WITNESS: It so seems to me.
THE DEFENSE: Do you have an opinion to a reasonable medical certainty?
THE WITNESS: I have. I think that the accident was due to—was caused by the illness under which Mr. [Wilson] was at that time involved in.

Dr. Salzman's testimony was given in terms less conclusory than those of Dr. Schultz. However, it became clear, as Dr. Salzman talked, that his knowledge of the defendant's recent past was haphazard and that his presentation often lacked organization and simplicity. His presentation, moreover, was marred both by his haste and his occasional staccato quality. When I asked him to "tell the court and the jury about the mental illness of the defendant, how it arose, developed and affected his mental and emotional processes, specifically on June 9, 1960," the response I received was this:

> Well, I could perhaps start with June ninth and then try to build up to this as best I can, and as *briefly* as I can:
> I believe that on June ninth, the situation which arose was the end result of a series of both delusional and what we call paranoid, meaning overwhelmingly frightened, attitudes that Mr. [Wilson] was undergoing, and when he was stopped and spoken to by one of the patrolmen, he got extremely frightened and sped off.
> Now, the reason I say this is because there is a great deal of data with regard to his having had an abnormal pathological delusional fear of policemen; he has been engaged in this particular kind of delusion for at least three years that I know, or maybe more, where he feels and felt that the policemen, particularly in No. 8 Precinct, were against him, were engaged in some plot to destroy him, to pin him up against the wall, as he puts it—.

The following interplay occurred between court, counsel and witness:

THE COURT: Are you getting all this from him?
THE WITNESS: Yes. Not all of it, most of this from him, some from a friend, a Mr. Rocca, who was a neighbor, information from his mother with regard to the expression of these ideas, and some from the social worker report, in which there is an abnormal exaggerated preoccupation, intense preoccupation with this whole problem of being the subject of abuse by policemen.
THE DEFENSE: Was there any real basis to this fear. Dr. Salzman?

THE WITNESS: Well, apparently not, because I was told by Mr. Rocca and by some of the No. 8 Precinct,[10] that actually some of them liked him; and I have raised this question on each interview with the prisoner, Mr. [Wilson], and cannot shake this notion at all. The fact is that there was not clearcut antagonism towards him; that there were some people at No. 8 who actually thought he was a fairly nice kid, as they put it.

So far as I can see, and as far as one can understand, there was no reasonable basis for these extreme feelings.

THE DEFENSE: Now, would you tell the court and the jury, Dr. Salzman, how—

THE WITNESS: Incidentally, I only wanted to mention one other incident which brought this out, and I did not mention:

That when he worked at the veterinarian's—and this was reported by the people on the staff there—he would see policemen across the street, people who were dressed in plainclothes, who he said were policemen, who he thought were watching him, were scrutinizing him, and while working at the veterinarian's he felt that his activities were watched. And shortly before June ninth he put his suits in various tailor's establishments, a rather peculiar business because he assumed that he was being trailed and he wanted to make sure that all his suits were not picked up, so he had his suits cleaned at three different establishments, and I never could understand why, except that, as he explains it, it was a way of fooling the cops who were trailing him.

It just came to my mind.

THE DEFENSE: Could you explain to the court and the jury,

---

[10] Dr. Salzman had at no time talked to any member at the No. 8 Precinct as he subsequently admitted. He interpreted his testimony as signifying only that he had been informed about the views of the No. 8 Precinct.

Dr. Salzman, how these . . . fears and fantasies originated?

THE WITNESS: Well, [to] the best of our knowledge, on the information that I have, most [of the fears and fantasies developed during] the early years of his life. I could only give you a sketch of the later years. But in the early years there was an extremely disrupted family situation.

There was an extreme amount of neglect in the home. The mother worked, the father presumably took care of the child.

He was a heavy drinker, and there was a great deal of evidence that he rarely changed or even fed the child. This was translated into a great many pathological items of behavior then; headbanging, bed-rocking, sleepless activities, dietary problems, and so forth, and particularly in the first year—

THE DEFENSE: Dr. Salzman, if I may interrupt, would you describe to the court and the jury just what took place during that one year in more detail? You refer to headbanging and bed-rocking. What do you mean by these particular remarks and what is their significance in the first year of a child's development?

THE WITNESS: Well, the first year of the child's development is characterized by a total dependence upon the parents. The infant cannot take care of its needs in any regard and requires the good will of the parents.

When this is lacking, or if it is indifferent or even deliberately neglectful, you get various responses in the child towards this.

Some children may not survive it but when they do they develop a variety of symptoms which are indicative of abnormal situations. One of them is the headbanging in which the infant—the reasons why the infant does it are not very clear, but they are a response to a distressful situation inside—bangs its head against the side of the crib, floor, wherever it is, rather extensive banging, so that you get black and blue marks.

There are exaggerated movements—physical movements—in what is known as rocking, in which the infant will bounce back and forth in its crib. It's an expression of excited neurological symptomatology. There are some dietary problems which are rather common and understandable, and the bed-wetting, which was not present then but which came later, which extended to the eighth year, was another sort of auxiliary fact about the extreme situation that this infant was undergoing.

When asked to describe "the personality of this boy," Dr. Salzman replied:

> I see this young man as somebody who is extremely sullen, overwhelmed with anger and resentments, a person who presents a picture of a frightened sort of animal-like individual who feels [the] pressure of an unfriendly world, with antagonisms all around him, with inability to trust anybody, to feel close, and to feel that anyone is safe to be with, and underneath this, interestingly enough, when you do get to know him, in some ways he is rather a warm boy.
>
> This does not seem contradictory if you get to know him a little better, of a frightened little boy, rather than someone who is angry as he appears on the surface.
>
> Now, the picture of him essentially is someone who is being hounded, tormented, trailed and constantly endangered. . . .

The direct examination of Dr. Salzman was concluded by asking whether the St. Elizabeths Hospital records which he had studied reflected "an attempt at psychodynamic investigation. . . ."

His answer was: "No, not the *records*."

I was forced to inquire: "What does?"

Dr. Salzman replied: "The *records* do not."

Since it seemed clear that the case of the defendant would be gravely damaged by the testimony of the St. Elizabeths Hospital physicians representing the official view of that hospital and one based upon essentially descriptive psychiatric thinking, I attempted to stress the theme of a lack of evidence of psychodynamic examination at St. Elizabeths. Dr. Salzman, it will be recalled, had furnished an affidavit in the Bradley case that adequate psychiatric examinations in court cases could be conducted "only by intensive psychoanalytic techniques." I now asked him upon redirect if it were ". . . possible for a psychiatrist to determine the origin of the illness, how it arose, developed, and affected the mental and emotional processes of the defendant, without significant training in psychoanalysis?" Dr. Salzman retorted:

> Well, that's a different question and I think there we have a matter of definition because the area is confused. The training of psychiatrists today includes such a background in what we call psychoanalytic techniques and methodology that it is hard to separate what is psychiatric and what is psychoanalytic, and I am not sure that that is particularly profitable.
>
> What is significant is that the skill in exploration that comes from these techniques in doing psychodynamic investigations, are what we call psychoanalytic. That is where they came from.

I persisted. I inquired as to whether he knew of a single fully-qualified psychoanalyst on the staff of St. Elizabeths Hospital. Dr. Salzman replied that he did not know the *entire* staff. I then asked him if the records of St. Elizabeths reflected an attempt at psychoanalytic investigation. Before the witness could reply, the court stated, "I don't think you have to have a psychoanalytic investigation to determine a man's sanity and I think the Doctor agrees with that." This, in essence, was Dr. Salzman's position.

The concluding part of Dr. Salzman's testimony seriously undermined the basic position of the defense—which was that no adequate psychodynamic investigation had taken place at St. Elizabeths Hospital.[11] The need for surrebuttal

---

[11] A behavioral scientist, observing the trial for another N.I.H. project, saw the matter with even greater pessimism. In his view, this part of the Salzman testimony, had "torpedoed the defendant's case."

witnesses at the end of the prosecution's case seemed imperative.

THE SECOND DAY OF THE TRIAL

Dr. James A. Ryan was the first expert witness for the defense upon the resumption of the trial. He was the youngest of the defense doctors; he had not yet been certified as a specialist by the American Board of Psychiatry and Neurology; nor had he, unlike the two witnesses who preceded him, completed his psychoanalytic training.

He had examined the defendant on two separate occasions prior to the trial. He had taken the initiative in seeking out the defendant again on the day of his testimony and interviewing him briefly that morning.

He had studied the records which I had made available to him and had "talked with . . . [the defendant's] mother on the telephone for a period of about half an hour . . . [and] with one of his neighbors, Mr. Rocca, for a period of about five minutes."

His handling of legally critical questions was, unlike that of the preceding witnesses, articulate, grammatical and direct, and his teamwork with defense counsel gratifying.

THE DEFENSE: Based upon your examination and study of this case, Doctor Ryan, do you have an opinion, to a reasonable medical certainty as to whether the defendant, Walter X. Wilson, was suffering from a mental disease on June 9, 1960?
THE WITNESS: Yes, I do.
THE DEFENSE: And would you tell the court and jury what that opinion is, please?
THE WITNESS: In my opinion he was then suffering from a major mental disease, one which profoundly affected his judgment and his ability to moderate and guide his own behavior.

THE DEFENSE: Doctor Ryan, did you also form an opinion to a reasonable medical certainty as to whether the events charged in the indictment were the products of the mental illness in question?

THE WITNESS: Yes, I did.

THE DEFENSE: And what is your opinion, sir?

THE WITNESS: In my opinion the events prior to [those with] which Mr. [Wilson] has been charged were the direct product of a major mental illness.

THE DEFENSE: And what is the name of the major mental illness, Dr. Ryan?

THE WITNESS: At the time of the crimes with which he is charged, I believe he was suffering from an acute episode of paranoid schizophrenia. Perhaps a name that would designate it a little more accurately would be a schizophrenic panic reaction.

Dr. Ryan maintained easy rapport with the courtroom audience, sensing the points most likely to prove of interest to his lay listeners and discussing them in his portraiture of his patient.

Asked as to how long the basic schizophrenic process had existed, Dr. Ryan provided the following account, interrupted by an occasional question:

THE WITNESS: I believe that it has existed for at least five years going back to the time of his prior admission to the D.C. General Hospital, and I believe that it is still existing even at the present time.

THE DEFENSE: Would you tell us something about that disease process and how it manifests itself?

THE WITNESS: This is describing the more chronic disease condition which I found which I would call a chronic state of paranoid schizophrenia in distinction from the condition at the time of the crime, acute panic reaction: the more chronic illness was manifested to me at the time of my examination by basically two findings; one was that there was evidence of delusions of persecution. These involved largely people in the police department who were, he felt, out to get him.

I might say that in arriving at a conclusion that he had such delusions, I had to make a distinction, which we often have to make, between a person who would be a "cop hater"—we many times have to examine a patient who has a rather fixed resentment about the police—but because of the very extensive nature of Mr. [Wilson's] fears about the police, I have concluded that he has delusions of persecution even at the present time.

If I might, while discussing the presence of delusions of persecution, there were other evidences of this type of delusion. For example, in my examination of Mr. [Wilson] on Friday, after the trial had been on for one day, he spontaneously began the interview by saying that he was going to get a certain individual, he was going to strangle him, if this individual came in court again he might jump up and try to choke him.

I asked him to tell me more about this, and he said it was that person, he used an epithet, called him an 'S.O.B.,' that man was against him; and I asked him who the man was, and he said it was a man—at this point he explained that they had asked before picking the jury if any of the jury had any reason of prejudice, and reason not to be on the jury, and that this one person had said yes, he did have a reason not to be on the jury and that this man was prejudiced against him, and if he could get hold of this one individual who admitted in court he was prejudiced, he would kill him.

By way of pointing up how there is a delusion involved here, I then explained to him that this is a procedure which is designed to protect him. Persons who might have any reasons to be against him are screened out in this way at court, and that this person apparently had some reason not to be on the jury and that actually then this person was someone who was acting in his best interests.

At this point he said, "Well, I still want to get him, but it's those other people who are on the jury. He is the only one who admitted it. The others are all there to get me, and they were put there by the Number 8 Police Department."

This actually came out a little later about the Number 8 Police Department, so his feeling was that the whole jury was rigged and this one individual who he wanted to kill was another person who was in a plot against him, so in this way his idea about getting back at a person who seemed to be acting in his best interests becomes logical in a morbid way; becomes logical because he felt that this person was just part of a whole plot of people to hurt him.

THE DEFENSE: Is it possible, Doctor Ryan, that these unusual statements on the part of the defendant may be the product of an inherently bad person rather than a sick person?

THE WITNESS: I would say that this type of thinking is an indication of a profound mental disorder.

Nor did Dr. Ryan, unlike the doctors who preceded him, lose sight of the appearance of his patient at the counsel table as he provided a narrative account of the dynamics of his patient's mental illness. Asked as to whether there were any "overt symptoms which . . . [were] easily noticeable about the defendant and which . . . [exemplified] his illness at this time," Dr. Ryan replied as follows:

Yes, there are.

As matter of fact, at this time—even at the present time—I believe the defendant is exhibiting a symptom of rocking which I had occasion to observe in the jail. This is not in itself a symptom of psychosis, but it is a symptom which has a long past history in his case.

As the witness made these remarks, judge and jury turned in the direction of Walter X. Wilson, who was rocking back and forth in his chair. Only after the judge and the jury had had an adequate opportunity to absorb this sight did Dr. Ryan resume his testimony. Dr. Ryan did not appear to be in any way striving for any dramatic effect. Walter's rocking back and forth in his chair at that specific moment was in fact all-absorbing both to the doctor, and to the judge and jury.

Dr. Ryan then went on to explain:

> Actually, he has a past history of headbanging. Up until he was about two years old he would bang his head against the side of the crib. This type of symptom, when it goes on for some period of time, in itself usually indicates a profound emotional turmoil on the part of a young child.
>
> Nowadays we see this particular symptom as a reason for a psychiatric referral even in a year old youngster.
>
> Following the period in which he had the symptom of headbanging he developed a symptom of rolling or rocking which is another very profound indication of emotional unrest in a youngster. He developed this symptom at age three and it has continued on up until the present time.
>
> Now, this is a symptom in which a person adopts a rocking motion. Basically, they may use it at bedtime; most commonly they use it at bedtime to get to sleep at night. Psychologically we believe that it is based on the rocking motion of a cradle. There is something in the general rocking motion that may help a severely disturbed person to get to sleep.
>
> Now, during the course of my examination at the jail this symptom became a sign, that is, it became something objective which I was able to observe, and it came on about midway through my first interview with Mr. [Wilson] at a time when we were talking about his

mother, when he spontaneously began to rock back and forth.

I suggest that perhaps this sign may be present right now. I would say that this is just a little bit of what I actually observed in the way of rocking at jail. At the jail the rocking was quite profound, involved his whole body, actually, rocking back and forth without an apparent awareness on his part that he was rocking. It continued for perhaps twenty minutes or so while we were talking about matters that he was then distressed about.

THE DEFENSE: Can you tell us about any of the other symptoms of his illness?

THE WITNESS: Yes. There was one other indication, major indication, of illness.

There is one other classical manifestation of this disease which we speak of as flatness, or flattening of the mood.

Now, flattening of the mood is something which a psychiatrist is specially trained to observe. In order to explain how I saw this symptom I would have to explain what we mean by the mood.

You know normally people show variations in their mood. You know that you may meet a person and say that person is a very warm individual, or you may speak of someone as being very spontaneous or full of life or vibrant personality. These are laymen's comments on the mood of another person. Similarly, you might meet an individual and say, 'Well, that person is a cold fish, he hardly cracked a smile all the time I was with him.' These both are comments on a person's mood.

Now, the normal variations in mood can be very subtle and a psychiatrist is specially trained to see subtle variations in the mood.

The mood actually reflects a person's interest in his surroundings, in response to things that are happening in—for example, in a discussion with a doctor a patient's mood normally varies up and down, may become a little angry, or may become warm hearted, may feel good, may show pleasure in the course of a discussion with the doctor, and these are normal mood variations.

Now, in Mr. [Wilson's] case throughout the first twenty minutes in which I saw him I would say that he showed a flattening of the mood, that is, he was talking about himself, he was responding to questions, but with no variation whatsoever in his mood. A little bit of variation began to come in after he developed the rocking motion. Then after that there was an indication of very hostile mood, and then, finally, at the close of my talk with him there was a little evidence of warmth, a reaching out to me for some kind of interest in him. This only came at the end of an hour and fifteen minute discussion with him. So that at the start there was a sustained period in which he displayed flattening of the mood, and flattening of the mood does indicate a person who has withdrawn his interests from his surroundings and pulled into himself in a very serious way, something which is only seen in the presence of a major mental illness such as schizophrenia.

We have evidence that the illness existed five years ago, I would say very clear evidence in the records of D.C. General Hospital in reports of doctors who at that time found flatness of affect. Two of my colleagues on the staff, Doctor Schultz and Doctor Costa, at that time made the same observation about the mood which I had occasion to make last week. Also the thinking disorder is indicated in the record at that time so that it is an illness that was present as far back as five years ago.

Now, how an illness like this actually gets started is a matter of . . . [dispute]. For example, there are schools of psychiatry that would say this illness has a chemical origin, and there are other schools of psychiatry that say no, it has a psychological origin. I believe that the predominant psychiatric theory about an illness like this would say that there are undoubtedly psychological factors even though there may be chemical influences.

Now, the kind of psychological factors that would appear to be involved in the origin of this illness were obtained in the history which I got from Mrs. [Wilson]. She related that . . . very early in his life it was necessary for her to turn her attention from her son to work, that even before he was born she was having serious trouble with her husband, that her husband had been an alcoholic for a number of years, that he beat her up, and in characteristic fashion of a person who would have a serious drinking problem her husband had extra trouble in tolerating her pregnancy with [Walter]. So that she herself had a considerable background of reasons to have worry about having her son in the first place, worrying about giving birth to him.

And then shortly after birth she continued to have trouble by way of fights with her husband. He actually moved out, I believe, shortly after the time of [Walter's] birth, and he came and went for a period of several years. Now, his coming and going again was marked at all time by episodes of violence between Mr. and Mrs. [Wilson].

This kind of violence can't exist in the life of a youngster without raising the possibility of having a serious illness. Now, I am not saying that every youngster who is exposed to violence has a serious illness. Many of them have ways of compensating so that the illness does not develop, but when we see this history and the coming and going, the insecurity created by absence of the father from the home, the insecurity created by violence which the youngster experiences, then we see at least a strong, early sort of fertilizing process that may make a way for major mental illness.

Now, I have already touched on the indications of serious emotional turmoil early in life; the symptom of headbanging which existed for, I believe, about a year and a half, just roughly age two to three and a half, is a very serious symptom, one for which we would always at this time advise psychiatric evaluation, again, not necessarily an indication that schizophrenia is then present, but an indication of serious emotional turmoil.

The subsequent symptoms of rocking before going to bed at night is a very profound pathological sign, and then there is further history of this child being difficult. Often we believe the origins of the illness do go well back into childhood, and they are described by parents as a difficult child, one that didn't get along with other children, one that kept to himself more.[12]

There is indication that the illness may have been present in the period . . . when [Walter] was about eight and had acquired a collection of knives and had threatened to use one of the knives on his father if his father ever came back. This would suggest, even at that time, a very deep feeling of insecurity and a tendency to have homicidal impulses, a youngster who would carry a knife at that age and speak of using a knife on his father, so that it is difficult to say when the illness actually arose. It appears to have been present five years ago. There are indications that there was a severe degree of emotional unrest going back to age one and a half or two.

THE DEFENSE: Now, Doctor Ryan, do you have an opinion as to the mental and emotional processes of the defendant [Walter X. Wilson], on June 9, 1960, and the

---

[12] The words in the official trial transcript are "different child." It is obvious that this is one of the stenographical or typographical errors which marks many a page of an average transcript. I have taken the liberty of recapturing what I believe to be the true meaning by substituting the obvious.

effect of those mental and emotional processes upon the events of that day?

THE WITNESS: Yes, I do.

THE DEFENSE: And would you give us the benefit of your opinion, please?

THE WITNESS: I believe that on that day Mr. [Wilson], who was then chronically ill, [with the] same illness I have described, suffered a worsening of his illness. As far as I can see there were two things involved, two factors involved in the worsening of his illness.

For one thing, from a psychological point of view, there had been a worsening because he had hoped to get into the service and he had talked with Mr. Rocca, his neighbor, about his disappointments in actually trying to get into the service, but two other factors appeared to bring on an acute worsening on the evening of June 9.

One of these factors was that Mr. [Wilson] had taken five tranquilizing pills at approximately nine o'clock in the evening and the other one was that about two hours after that—

THE COURT: How do you know?

THE WITNESS: This is the history, Your Honor. I don't know for a certainty.

THE COURT: Who told you that?

THE WITNESS: This is history that I obtained from Mr. [Wilson].

THE COURT: He told you that he took five tranquilizing pills?

THE WITNESS: Yes, Your Honor.

THE COURT: What kind?

THE WITNESS: These tranquilizing pills were dog tranquilizers which he said he obtained from—I believe it is the Edgemoor Animal Hospital where he had been employed some months before.

THE COURT: They give tranquilizers to dogs?

THE WITNESS: Yes, Your Honor, they do.

THE COURT: Even a dog is nervous and has to have tranquilizers? What do they give them?
THE WITNESS: This particular tranquilizer is made up of about four different ingredients.
THE COURT: Does it have a name?
THE WITNESS: I don't know the trade name, Your Honor.
THE COURT: Well, is it similar to Equanil, Miltown, or Thorazine, or something like that?
THE WITNESS: Yes, it is similar to them. It has actually the same ingredients used in human tranquilizers. This one has some phenobarbital in it and it has one of the newer tranquilizers mephenesin in it, and I believe it has bromide in it as well. I am not sure what the fourth ingredient is.
THE COURT: He took five of these on the date in question at about what time?
THE WITNESS: At about nine o'clock, Your Honor.
THE COURT: How strong are these?
THE WITNESS: This would be difficult to actually know because it is not a preparation used in regular medical practice, but from the amount of ingredients that were present, the recognizable ingredients that are in the tranquilizers, I would say five of them plus a later history of drinking nine beers would create a good possibility for a toxic reaction, a drug state.

Dr. Ryan then proceeded to discuss another symptom of the defendant's illness:

One element in his illness has been an enormous fear of being attacked or being hurt, and mixed together with the fear of being attacked is a fear of being approached by another man for a—what we would call a homosexual situation. These are two fears, and two separate fears which are very strong in the background of the patient. They would be so great that at the time of my last interview the patient brought out that he couldn't stand having a marshal sit behind him; he wondered, "why can't that man sit in front of me where I can see him." So this is a burden that he carries with him, I would say, at all times, his fear of another man attacking him; and then side by side with that is fear of another man approaching him and trying to have some form of sexual play with him.

Now, these two fears are...present. I have to point them up because they are so vital to the understanding [of] the disturbed state in which I felt he entered on this evening.

These fears are so great that he has frequent dreams of men chasing him, he has had dreams of men approaching him, has dreams in which he murders men who approach him, he has had dreams in which his father is one of the men who approaches him and tries to engage him in activity, and sometimes the outcome of the dreams is that he falls down a cliff or falls over a steep building. These dreams have been regularly present for a very long time.

Both the witness and defense counsel were side-tracked at this particular stage from pursuing the theme of the panic reaction brought about by the approach of a homosexual to the defendant as a result of a skeptical and digressive series of judicial questions as to the significance of dream interpretation in psychiatric diagnosis. However, Dr. Ryan picked up the threads of his testimony on direct examination with these remarks:

I might mention one further observation about the fear which would go into this, which would be another element, in my mind, regarding his fear of attack. It came out in my second interview on Friday, something which I suspected after my first interview, this patient has been having auditory hallucinations of a threatening nature. He has been hearing voices which tell him that someone is going to attack him, also voices which call him bad names. He has been hearing these for about five years.

I say that I suspected it after my first interview because—I might say, there is an art to learning that a patient has this degree of illness, that they have a hallucination, and there is a proper time for bringing the question in. Many patients are ashamed of the fact that they hear voices that threaten them and they won't tell you.

In my first examination when it came to a point where I did ask a question about hearing voices the patient dodged the question, he didn't answer it, but he went off and began to talk about dreams which he had had.

This is something that often happens in a patient who has hallucinations. A patient who is not having hallucinations will answer the question very quickly and very directly that they are not hearing voices.

In the second interview with him at a point later in the interview he finally confessed to me, as it were, that he had been hearing voices in the evening, which is a characteristic time for hearing them, at the end of the day just before going to bed or while in bed when it was quiet, when his interest from his surroundings was fully withdrawn, that he had been hearing voices, and he felt very ashamed about hearing them, he felt bad because the voices called him very bad names, and also he had always been worried because these voices threatened him.

Dr. Ryan then added that Walter Wilson needed treatment in a maximum security ward of a mental hospital for a long period of time and that at the present time he was both homicidal and suicidal.

Cross-examination largely confirmed the strength of Dr. Ryan's direct testimony.

THE PROSECUTION: This stress that you spoke of in direct examination, wasn't that in reference to the police car coming up on the defendant, and things of that sort?

THE WITNESS: In my analysis of the case I see actually two stresses; the initial stress would have to do with the feeling on the defendant's part that he had—that he was being approached by another man for an immoral act.

. . . .

THE PROSECUTION: The acute reaction you speak of is a reaction to the homosexual advance, be it real or imaginary?

THE WITNESS: Yes, that's correct.

THE PROSECUTION: How is that associated with the police coming upon the scene?

THE WITNESS: Again, behind this fear is a fear of attack, and there is evidence that he has had a long standing fear of attack, that I would believe to be a delusional fear of attack from police.

THE PROSECUTION: How about the delusional fear of attacks from homosexuals?

THE WITNESS: Yes, this has also been present.

THE PROSECUTION: But actually if there was an approach by a homosexual it would not have been a delusion.

THE WITNESS: No. Again the approach may not have been a delusion, but the persistent feeling that people around him were trying to engage him in immoral acts, this is the delusion; this is present still.

THE PROSECUTION: That is as regards these other people, but we are saying that the acute reaction was this one homosexual approaching him on that night; isn't that correct?

THE WITNESS: Yes, in this particular instance.

THE PROSECUTION: And he had some fear of that individual homosexual; right?

THE WITNESS: Well, again, whether he had a real fear of the individual or whether he had a misperceived fear of the individual, he still had a chronic delusion that men would try to engage him in homosexual behavior.

THE PROSECUTION: Well, the chronic delusion, did that exist on June eighth?

THE WITNESS: Yes, I would say that it did.

THE PROSECUTION: How did this condition on June eighth vary from that on June ninth?

THE WITNESS: I would say that the delusion has been present for many years and is still present.

Fortunately, at this point, the line of cross-examination pursued by prosecuting counsel picked up the theme of the panic reaction brought about by the approach of the homosexual to the defendant on the day of the accident and permitted Dr. Ryan to put it in clear perspective in his testimony.

THE PROSECUTION: How about the acute reaction; was there acute reaction on June 8?

THE WITNESS: On the day of the—

THE PROSECUTION: The day before.

THE WITNESS: The day before.
   Again, the predisposition to an acute reaction was undoubtedly there, but he needed something to set it off.

THE PROSECUTION: What set it off on June 9?

THE WITNESS: Again, I would say that it was either a real approach or it was the mere circumstance of being in the car along with another man.

THE PROSECUTION: You know that he was in the car with another man?

THE WITNESS: Again, this is a history as I have obtained it from Mr. [Wilson].

THE PROSECUTION: Did you determine who the owner of the car was on that particular night?

THE WITNESS: No, I don't know the owner's identity.

THE PROSECUTION: And what about the—immediately after

this homosexual experience, be it real or imaginary, being an offer of actual fulfillment of the act, what was the defendant's reaction?

THE WITNESS: The immediate reaction is one of fear followed by a breakthrough of angry impulse which he described as 'seeing red,' and 'going to pieces,' followed by a panic and a need to get away.

THE PROSECUTION: How did he manifest that panic and that fear to get away; what did he do?

THE WITNESS: Then he began to kick and thrash about in the car, punch at the other man who was in the car, finally kick him out of the car. He said at first, 'Maybe I drove over him, maybe I didn't; I had to get away.'

THE PROSECUTION: And then did he drive away?

THE WITNESS: He then drove away.

THE PROSECUTION: And then what happened?

THE WITNESS: After that, my impression is that his recollections are somewhat blurred, but there did come a time when he saw a flashing red light.

THE PROSECUTION: What happened then?

THE WITNESS: Then there was further panic—further, I would say an increasing state of panic at the thought that the police were after him, again based on a long standing fear of what police might do to him.

I concluded my questioning of the witness on redirect examination by inquiring as to whether he believed Walter Wilson to be subject to commitment to a mental hospital even if he were to assume that no crime had been committed by him in this case. There was immediate objection by the government.

The emerging judicial attitude toward the question of Walter's mental health was then promptly portrayed in these responses:

THE COURT: Overruled. He has schizophrenia, hasn't he?
THE WITNESS: Yes, Your Honor. Not every patient who has

schizophrenia is committed to a mental institution. I would have to become more specific, if I may—

THE COURT: What type is that?

THE WITNESS: Right at the present time it is paranoid schizophrenia.

THE COURT: You say that if you are a paranoid schizophrenic you shouldn't be committed?

THE WITNESS: No. We do recognize such a thing as a chronic paranoid schizophrenic who, we may feel, is not dangerous to other people.

THE COURT: I am not talking about other people; I am talking about this person. You said he was dangerous, didn't you?

THE WITNESS: Yes, Your Honor.

THE COURT: The question now is, even if he hadn't committed this crime should he be committed to a mental hospital.

THE WITNESS: Yes, Your Honor. Based on my present examination I would say he should be committed to a mental institution.

On recross-examination, prosecuting counsel sought to inquire of Dr. Ryan as to what "stage" the defendant's illness had progressed.

Once again the court intervened, clearly showing its belief in the defendant's mental illness. "You say that he has had it for five years. . . . That wouldn't be an early stage, would it?"

THE THIRD DAY OF THE TRIAL

I assumed that the jury had been deluged with enough psychiatric testimony for the moment and decided upon a change of pace.

The next two witnesses I called, therefore, were laymen who had known the defendant. The first was the night attendant at the Edgemoor Animal Hospital, at which the defendant had worked, who testified about Walter's suspicion and fear of being watched by the police. The second was the manager of a barbershop who had lived next door to the defendant. Approximately three months prior to the accident, this witness had made a point of befriending the defendant. He reported that the defendant had given his clothes to different cleaners because of his fear that they would be taken away from him. He further reported that the defendant had refused food that was offered to him and recounted that he had "observed on one particular occasion after offering him food, that . . . he went downstairs, reached into a bag of dog food, which is a dry substance mixed with water, and he got himself a handful of it." This witness concluded his testimony on an unexpected and dramatic note. I inquired: "Would you say . . . [that the defendant] was getting better or worse towards the end of your acquaintance?" He replied: "I would say worse, basing it on what transpired . . . he was getting worse, and I might add one thing: Walter's physical appearance at the present moment—he used to have jet black hair; it is no longer jet black."

This was the second time that a witness succeeded in directing all eyes upon Walter X. Wilson. As judge and jury turned to look at him, Walter was seen, his eyes fixed on the floor, rocking rhythmically in his chair. His hair was not jet black.

The next witness was Dr. Brigitte Julian, of St. Elizabeths hospital, the only medical member of the St. Elizabeths staff who had expressed a willingness to testify that the defendant was mentally ill. Dr. Julian had seen Walter Wilson at a diagnostic staff conference at St. Elizabeths and had reviewed the available information about him at that time.

She declared that the patient had not displayed any "flagrantly psychotic symptoms" at the conference. She expressed her opinion, nonetheless, that he was suffering from mental illness.

When asked by the court about the specific nature of the mental illness she diagnosed, she said that "the label . . . [she] would have put on it at that time would have been . . . an emotionally unstable personality."

When asked by the court whether anybody at the staff conference agreed with her, she replied: "I think they said he was partly sick but not sick enough to warrant diagnosis of mental illness—and I think this is where we disagreed."

She added, still under questioning by the court, that she thought ". . . that the majority of them felt that he was sick. . . . They expressed it in terms of his being incapable of functioning in the society and his being very impulsive, incapable of sufficient controls in minor stress situations. . . ."

In her view, the staff conference did not reach the conclusion that Walter Wilson was suffering from a mental disease or defect because "his deviation from the normal was not sufficient to warrant the diagnosis of mental disorder."

Dr. Julian expressed her opinion that the mental illness of the defendant had been in existence on June 9, 1960.

When asked by the court as to what she meant by the words "mentally ill," she replied:

> I think mental illness takes many forms, and I do not know whether I am expert enough to give you now a summary of those symptoms which are common in all mental illness, but I think that mentally ill people have more difficulty than others to deal with stress situations in life; they are usually inefficient, they can very easily be panicked. They might sometimes use ways of dealing with problems in their life which seem to be rather irrational; they don't seem to fit the purpose of what they try to achieve. They have a very short frustration tolerance. They might show physical symptoms of overt anxiety, of trembling, shaking and blocking of speech; these are only to name a few.

When the court pursued by inquiring as to what specific symptoms the defendant had, Dr. Julian replied:

> The way I saw him in the conference was, as I said before, I felt that some of his answers to questions showed very bad

judgment. I felt that he was preoccupied so that he could hardly tear himself away from his idea of hate, that he was very impulsive.

Significantly, Dr. Julian declared in answer to my question as to whether or not it was possible to rule out the existence of a psychotic episode on June 9, 1960 that it was not and "I don't think that anybody at St. Elizabeths Hospital would say that."

Cross-examination of Dr. Julian was essentially restricted to showing that she had not observed any flagrant psychotic symptomatology about her patient.

I attempted to conclude my redirect examination of the witness with a question designed to shed light upon the psychiatric policy of the St. Elizabeths staff which permitted it, as expressed by Dr. Julian, to find a given individual sick, but not sick enough, and hence to be diagnosed as without mental disorder.

THE DEFENSE: You said the St. Elizabeths' doctors at the staff conference thought that he was sick, but not sick enough. How do people happen to talk that way? I find it as difficult to follow as the court.

THE WITNESS: This is my own, completely my own opinion. I have been in John Howard Pavilion dealing with patients—

THE COURT: Answer the question. The question is very simple; there is nothing complicated about it. You said the staff conference was of the opinion that the man was—did you say mentally sick?

THE DEFENSE: Sick, but not sick enough; is that right?

THE WITNESS: Yes.

How is that possible, was that your question?

THE DEFENSE: Yes, Dr. Julian. Could you explain that to us?

THE WITNESS: My opinion is that most psychiatrists—very many psychiatrists, and particularly my colleagues—do think that people who act out against society are sick, and—

THE COURT: What is that again? Everybody that commits a crime is mentally sick?

THE WITNESS: Is sick, yes.

THE COURT: Do you believe that?

THE WITNESS: Yes.

THE COURT: You don't believe in free will, then?

THE WITNESS: I don't know what it is.

THE COURT: You don't know what free will is?

THE WITNESS: What do you mean by that?

THE COURT: Don't you understand what free will is? You are a psychiatrist and you don't know what I mean when I say free will?

THE WITNESS: No. I don't.

THE COURT: Don't I have a will of my own to do as I please?

THE WITNESS: Could you take a concrete example?

THE COURT: Suppose I want to go up to a movie this afternoon. I could go, couldn't I, if I chose to?

THE WITNESS: Yes.

THE COURT: I could go up and buy a suit of clothes or a hat. I could go to a football game. I could do any number of things. I could exercise the free will to do what I want to do. You never heard of free will before?

THE WITNESS: This is what you call free will?

THE COURT: What do you call it? Is there anything different? Isn't it a person's ability to make up his mind to do something?

THE WITNESS: I thought you wanted to know about a person's ability to make up their mind not to do something, which might be different.

THE COURT: That is free will; you have a will to do it or not to do it, don't you?

THE WITNESS: I think not in all cases, no.

THE COURT: When you said the staff conference concluded the man was sick, but wasn't sick enough, I assume that you meant by that that he was suffering from some mental deficiency.

THE WITNESS: From mental illness.

THE COURT: That is the same thing, isn't it?
THE WITNESS: Yes.

The court pursued its questioning of the witness with such zeal as to bring out in the presence of the jury and in clear violation of a statutory prohibition that the defendant had been found to be mentally competent to stand trial by St. Elizabeths Hospital.

An immediate motion for a mistrial, based upon the comment, was denied.[13] However, the court instructed the jury to disregard that remark.

Walter X. Wilson had for once been following the proceedings with keen interest. Although sporadically rocking in his chair, he fixed his eyes upon Dr. Julian whose testimony appeared all-absorbing to him. His restlessness, however, seemed to mount.

When I saw him briefly in the cell block during a recess prior to the resumption of Dr. Julian's testimony he was visibly agitated. He was pacing up and down, grasping the bars of the cell and shouting something like: "They lie. Why do they all lie?"

I felt at that time that I could very readily succeed in reassuring the boy. On one or two previous occasions, a reassuring comment made by me within the cell block had resulted in his seeming visibly relaxed and more "normal" in appearance at the counsel table.

While the case appeared to have been going well it seemed clear that whatever points had been scored by the defense in the courtroom had been based primarily upon a showing of psychotic as distinct from nonpsychotic psychopathology.

---

[13] *Cf.*, Horton v. United States, 317 F.2d 595 (D.C. Cir. 1963); for the underlying statutory enactment barring the disclosure to the jury of an accused's competency to stand trial see 18 U.S.C. §4244 (1949). The section provides *inter alia:*

"A finding by the judge that the accused is mentally competent to stand trial shall in no way prejudice the accused in a plea of insanity as a defense to the crime charged; such finding shall not be introduced in evidence on that issue nor otherwise be brought to the notice of the jury."

One remembers with ease in such a context the instances in which a skillful prosecutor had destroyed the claim of a psychotic illness by dwelling upon the defendant's appearance of 'normalcy' at the counsel table, and ascribing even pronounced manifestations of anxiety to 'normal' apprehension or a sense of guilt.[14]

It was my judgment at that time that the boy's rocking at the counsel table constituted in many ways evidence indispensable to the return of a verdict of not guilty by reason of insanity at the hands of an average jury, such as the one in the instant case. I deliberately desisted from providing any reassuring comments in response to the boy's increasing agitation.

Redirect examination was resumed subsequently and produced the following disclosures:

THE DEFENSE: Doctor Julian, do you know whether or not the diagnostic procedures used upon the defendant at St. Elizabeths would have been different had he been placed in, say, the Dix Pavilion rather than the John Howard Pavilion?
THE WITNESS: I don't think the procedures would have been different.
THE DEFENSE: What would have been different?
THE WITNESS: In what way and for what reason?
THE PROSECUTION: Your Honor, I object to this; it is immaterial.

---

[14] The following provides striking illustrative material. Mr. Hantman, Assistant U.S. Attorney, in his closing argument to the jury in United States v. Stewart, Crim. No. 633-53 (D.D.C. 1962), stated as follows:

"There is one real, important factor in this case that has not been discussed. You weigh, ladies and gentlemen, everything that the defense psychiatrists have told you about the illness this defendant has, and its severity and its degree and stack it up against the defendant's demeanor all four weeks he has been here.

If he was as sick as these doctors have indicated, you should have seen the demonstrations here."

Transcript of Proceedings, United States v. Stewart at 2204.

The Court: Well, I am interested in knowing why it would be different. You examine a patient—I don't care whether it is in a pavilion, Howard Hall, or where it is—if a psychiatrist reaches a conclusion—I am interested to hear the answer of this witness.

The Witness: I think that it would be different because of the fact that most of the patients in John Howard Pavilion have criminal charges, and I think that psychiatrists cannot completely disregard what this implicates that they have from the charges, and also cannot discard their court experience; and it is just my opinion, but I feel that many psychiatrists feel that they are not used as informants in court, but they are used as tools to kill the *Durham* rule in the District, and they are often made fools of, and that they are in some way—

The Court: What is this? Used as tools to kill the *Durham* rule; is that what you said?

The Witness: This is my impression.

The Court: What psychiatrists have been used to kill the *Durham* rule?

The Witness: I think this is a deduction some have drawn from the way they have been used in their position as expert witnesses.

The Court: Who?

The Witness: Colleagues of mine.

The Court: Who? What doctors, what psychiatrist had told you he is being used as a tool to kill the *Durham* rule?

The Witness: I didn't say they exactly said to me these words; this is my impression from talking to them about their court experience.

The Court: Who did you talk to?

The Witness: I have talked; for instance, have discussed cases like the one of [Walter Wilson] and others, where there was a dissenting opinion about whether the patient had or had not a mental disorder.

The Court: I am not concerned with that. All I want to know is what psychiatrists you talked to that gave you the impression they were used as tools in court to kill the *Durham* rule?

THE WITNESS: I think the physicians in the conference.

THE COURT: You got the impression after talking to Doctor Platkin and Doctor Read that they were being used as tools in court to kill the *Durham* rule; is that right?

THE WITNESS: Yes, but this is my formulation. They did not say that, I would like to state—

THE COURT: What did they say from which you got the impression?

THE WITNESS: They have said to me that they feel they are not used in order to give objective information, but their testimony is used to some extent to help the court make the decision which—

THE COURT: The court make the decision?

THE WITNESS: Let me say it this way: They feel that they are not basically used as informants. They say they are—

THE COURT: They say that they are used as informants?

THE WITNESS: No, that they are not used to give expert information only.

THE COURT: They are not used to give expert information. What are they used for?

THE WITNESS: I think that they think that their semantics and semantics here in court are very different.

THE COURT: I don't know what you're talking about. You mean my semantics and the doctors' are different?

THE WITNESS: Yes. And they feel that their information, that the questions they are asked are not asked in order so much to—it is not tried enough to understand what they are talking about.

THE COURT: Do you know that is a very serious statement you are making?

Are Doctor Platkin and Doctor Read here?

THE PROSECUTION: Not yet. Doctor Platkin is on call.

THE COURT: And Doctor Read?

THE PROSECUTION: I don't have Doctor Read.

THE COURT: Do you have him?
THE DEFENSE: No, Your Honor.
THE COURT: I want him.
   Now, in order to understand you correctly, you have had a conversation with Doctor Platkin and Doctor Read—
THE WITNESS: Yes,
THE COURT: —from which you gather the impression, from what they told you, that they were being used in court as tools to kill the *Durham* rule; is that your testimony?
THE WITNESS: Yes, that was my impression.

Diagnostic practices at St. Elizabeths Hospital, as described by Dr. Julian, had not been unsuspected by knowledgeable members of the Bar. This, however, in no way detracted from the startling quality of her testimony which was visibly disturbing to the legal members of the audience for differing reasons.

The next witnesses that day were psychologists, drawn from St. Elizabeths and D.C. General Hospitals respectively.

The Judge had in the past repeatedly expressed the view that psychologists were not properly qualified to testify as to the existence or nonexistence of mental illness. I had therefore prepared a memorandum of law designed to show the acceptability of psychological testimony in such cases and had filed it with the court preliminary to the calling of the first psychologist.[15]

The psychologists in this case furnished significant corroborative evidence of Walter Wilson's psychopathology.[16]

---

[15] This memorandum preceded the filing of the formal brief in support of the proposition upheld by the Court of Appeals, that psychologists were entitled to testify as to the existence or nonexistence of a mental illness in Jenkins v. United States, 307 F.2d 637 (D.C. Cir. 1962).

[16] A psychologist observing the case for another N.I.H. project reported as follows:
"The three psychologists who had tested the defendant in this particular case were all experienced and well-qualified clinical psychologists. Their test batteries overlapped considerably. Their test results and interpretations,
(Footnote continued on next page.)

Dr. Catherine Beardsley, the first psychologist to testify, had tested the defendant at St. Elizabeths in 1956. She described her role as a psychologist and the tests she had administered to the defendant.

THE DEFENSE: Doctor Beardsley, I understand you are a psychologist and not a psychiatrist.
THE WITNESS: I am a psychologist.
THE DEFENSE: Doctor Beardsley, would you inform us more specifically about your duties at St. Elizabeths Hospital?
THE WITNESS: Yes.

In my capacity as Director of Training in Psychology a major portion of my time is spent in the administration of the training program, of the Psychology trainees in the hospital. This involves, in addition to teaching duties and various other administrative duties, direct supervision, that is, work with the trainees in their diagnostic testing, that is, in their testing of patients, in their scoring of these tests, interpretation of these tests, and their writing them up to become an official part of the hospital record.

Other duties I have as a Clinical Psychologist include the testing of patients myself, the giving of complete psychological examination, scoring, analysis, and interpretation of these tests to the medical staff and other interested persons.

Another aspect of my work at the hospital is in the field of individual psychotherapy, working with individual patients as their therapist.

---

when heard, were very similar. This agrees with a finding of a preliminary questionnaire given to psychologists who have testified in court. 'Either psychologists tend to testify on the same side of the bar or their findings are not that discrepant.'"

Scheflen, *supra* note 8, at 333.

In my experience in the litigation of cases involving mental health I too have found the finding of psychologists in given instances to be markedly similar—in contrast to the findings of psychiatrists.

THE DEFENSE: Doctor Beardsley, could you tell us this: what is the role of the fully trained Clinical Psychologist in the field of mental examinations?

THE WITNESS: The fully trained Clinical Psychologist has, I would say, a three faceted role.

The major core of the Clinical Psychologist's training and his job as a professional person, the aspect of his training which makes him unique, is his ability in diagnostic testing, that is, in the making of complete personality studies of the person whom he tests.

His second function is that of therapist, psychotherapist.

And his third function is as a research person.

THE DEFENSE: Now, is this diagnostic testing which is done by the fully trained Clinical Psychologist accepted as part of a complete mental examination by contemporary psychiatry?

THE WITNESS: Yes.

THE DEFENSE: Doctor Beardsley, did there come a time in your duties at St. Elizabeths when you examined the defendant, [Walter X. Wilson]?

THE WITNESS: Yes.

THE DEFENSE: And would you tell the Court and jury how much time you spent with him in that examination?

THE WITNESS: May I refer to my notes?

I saw Mr. [Wilson] in February for a total of four sessions for testing. I would estimate a total time of between four and five hours.

THE DEFENSE: Would you tell the Court and jury what testing you engaged in?

THE WITNESS: Yes, I gave Mr. [Wilson] an intelligence test, standardized intelligence test for adults entitled the Wechsler Adult Intelligence Scale.

I administered to him two tests of memory, the Wechsler Memory Scale and the Benton Visual Retention Test. Then a test of concept formation entitled the Color Form Sorting; a test of visual motor co-ordination entitled the Bender-Gestalt, and three tests which are primarily thought of as personality tests, the Rorschach, the projective drawings, and the Szondi, spelled S-z-o-n-d-i.

THE DEFENSE: Would you tell us, Doctor Beardsley, what those tests revealed and what your interpretation of the test results were?

THE WITNESS: Yes.

THE COURT: Don't give the Szondi results because that is out in this court.

THE WITNESS: All right.

I will give only a general statement of my conclusions.

May I say this: that Mr. [Wilson] had been—I had available to me a battery of tests which had been administered by one of our psychologists to Mr. [Wilson] in 1956, and, therefore, my analysis was done in relation—had the advantage, actually, of being done in relation to the former test material.

I found in February a greater impairment in intellectual functioning now than we had found in 1956. I would like to explain that a little bit.

Ordinarily a so-called average person, when he takes one of these standardized tests which has many parts to it, gets a score which is approximately equal on all of these subtests. I found in Mr. [Wilson's] case that he was responding in a very erratic way. In some tests he could do very well; in some tests he could not do very well at all.

I found this to be more marked now than in the earlier set of test material. I found further a kind of thinking which we would not expect in a person of Mr. [Wilson's] potentially average intelligence. It is the kind of thinking which we call concrete or functional.

If I may give an example, that is, if I were to ask someone in what way an orange and a banana were alike, some might say, well, you eat them both, or someone might say they are both fruit.

THE COURT: That is one of the questions in the examination, isn't it?

THE WITNESS: Yes.

I do not know what Mr. [Wilson] responded to that question, but, in general, the type of thinking I found in many of his responses was of the simpler kind, that is, the kind by function, by what you do rather than by a more complex general statement.

I found also that he showed a good ability to tell what ought to be done in every day situations, but when put into a situation where he had to actually make application of these judgments, he did very poorly.

THE COURT: I thought you wanted the results of these tests.

THE DEFENSE: Yes, Your Honor, I did ask for results of these tests and the doctor's interpretation of these results.

THE COURT: I would like to have the results of the tests first.

THE WITNESS: You mean you would like to have an IQ?

THE COURT: What you say the results of the tests are; I don't know.

THE WITNESS: These are the results and my interpretation of the results constitute, actually, the results. The intelligence quotient, full scale intelligence quotient, was 77.

. . . .

THE DEFENSE: Had this gone up or down since the last psychological examination?

THE WITNESS: Down.

THE COURT: 77; is that borderline?

THE WITNESS: Yes.

THE COURT: All right.

THE WITNESS: It had come down from 90, which is low average. And what I was describing was the—what I call the pattern of his response which would give us the background of what I was calling his erratic or uneven behavior.

The memory quotient, which is parallel to an intelligence quotient, was consistent with the intelligence quotient and was 79. We interpret that in the similar fashion, and, as I say, the—I interpret the difference between the two sets of tests to be due to a greater variability in his functioning, to less ability to think as clearly and to express himself as well as he did earlier.

Personality tests revealed a severe state of anxiety, more than we saw in 1956. It was the kind of anxiety which we find, in this boy, associated with an actual fear that his feelings, particularly his less pleasant feelings, will burst out in action before he has a chance to control them. When a person is in this state of fear it is a kind of fear which we sometimes think of as almost panic.

I also saw in the test material an attempt to try to do something about this feeling of fear, and so much energy, that is, thinking in all of his waking hours, so much energy, going into trying to protect himself against these fears that he had very little left for appropriate behavior and relationship to the outside world.

I also found a tendency in this boy to not be able to tolerate his own feelings or to be able to see in himself what he really was thinking and feeling and, hence, the necessity for finding the blame for what he did or what he might do on the outside world. This is what we call projection; that is the technical term for it.

One of the ways in which this person tried to cope with this fear of the outbreak, of his emotions and his impulses, was to run blindly away from an immediate situation. We have here a personality—may I interrupt a moment here to go back to the so-called average person, the functioning person. Ordinarily, our emotional life, our emotions and our intelligence work pretty well together in the personality. Sometimes we become a little disabled by too strong emotions or situations arising from strong emotions, but ordinarily the average person can manage to go along.

The thing which I found reflected in the tests of Mr. [Wilson] was a failure of emotions and intelligence to be integrated in the way in which we expect them to be personalitywise in a person who functions within the average range.

Now, this failure of integration—rather, this pattern, let me say, of failure of integration, of sometimes in his thinking rather peculiar answers, rather peculiar thoughts coming out, this tremendous struggle and anxiety led me to the conclusion that this boy could have a definite break with reality.

I would say that those were my major conclusions on the basis of the test material.

. . .

THE DEFENSE: Doctor Beardsley, do you have a psychological opinion as to whether the incapacitating factors which you have described existed on June 9, 1960?
THE WITNESS: In my opinion they did.
THE DEFENSE: Thank you very much, Doctor Beardsley.

Cross examination essentially attempted to convey the point that the psychologist, like a laboratory technician, had no significant function beyond that of conveying his data to the psychiatrist whose judgment was to be regarded as both final and authoritative on all counts. The following is characteristic:

THE PROSECUTION: The answers to all of these tests and the impressions you conveyed to the psychiatrist; is that correct?
THE WITNESS: I did.
THE PROSECUTION: So that the psychiatrist, with all of his personal observations and the like, can make a determi-

tion and diagnosis of the man and can properly treat him; is that right?

THE WITNESS: That's right.

THE PROSECUTION: Nothing further.

Dr. Bernard I. Levy, Chief Psychologist of the D.C. General Hospital, was the next psychological expert called by the defense. Like Dr. Ryan, he sought out Walter Wilson during recesses and expressed concern as to the effect of the stress of the trial on his illness. To a greater extent than Doctor Beardsley, he was handicapped, albeit not critically, by the Court's view that a psychologist represented some lesser form of expertise. Doctor Levy based his testimony on both clinical interviewing and psychological testing:

THE DEFENSE: Did there come a time in the course of your duties at D.C. General Hospital when you had occasion to interview and examine the defendant, [Walter X. Wilson]?

THE WITNESS: Yes.

THE DEFENSE: And would you tell us what this examination consisted of?

THE WITNESS: The duration of the examination was approximately two hours. The first part of the examination was a clinical interview.

THE DEFENSE: Would you tell us what a clinical interview is, Doctor Levy?

THE WITNESS: It is an attempt, in sitting with a patient and using a variety of fairly complex techniques, to attempt to understand—first, to make friends with the patient because this is absolutely essential, and then to try to understand as much as it is possible of his difficulties and problems.

The type of interview I personally conduct is relatively flexible. There are interviewers who will conduct a rather rigid interview.

THE DEFENSE: Is it possible, Doctor Levy, to conduct an

interview in good faith and still fail to obtain any significant results because of the failure to establish the friendly contact which I believe you explained to be vital in this case?

THE WITNESS: It is my opinion that this is a relatively frequent problem with people who are not as experienced in interviewing, or under very unusual circumstances.

THE DEFENSE: Doctor Levy, isn't it possible that you might get a very experienced psychiatric interviewer, a highly competent man, who might not succeed in eliciting certain materials for evaluation of the patient?

THE PROSECUTION: He said psychiatric interviewer.
This doctor is psychological—

THE COURT: I will sustain the objection.

THE DEFENSE: May I amend it, by simply saying interviewer, subject to the Court's permission.

Is it possible that a skillful interviewer might occasionally fail to elicit vital data on the nature of an individual's illness?

THE WITNESS: Yes.

THE DEFENSE: What is essential, then, to the interview is the friendly contact, the rapport. Did you have that friendly contact and rapport?

THE WITNESS: It is virtually impossible to know for certain, but after several years of experience the clinician does get a feeling about the level of friendliness that exists, and I felt that it was sufficient at the time that I saw the defendant to conduct the interview.

THE DEFENSE: In addition to the clinical interview you conducted a number of tests, did you not?

THE WITNESS: Yes, a brief battery of tests.

THE DEFENSE: Would you tell the Court and the jury what those tests were?

THE WITNESS: The Rorschach, which is sometimes called the ink blot test, and a test called the Human Figure Drawings.

THE DEFENSE: Now, would you report to the Court and the jury first on the results of your clinical interview and tests and, second, upon your interpretation of those results.

THE WITNESS: I entered the meeting with the defendant expecting some amount of resistance from the defendant because this is fairly common. I was quite startled early in the interview when the defendant said something that made me pick up my ears. He said in a rather low and intense voice that he doesn't deserve all of this, and I decided at that moment to pursue that particular issue rather than something else, and he told me that he did not deserve the treatment, the good treatment he was receiving, the excellent lawyer he had, and the consideration that he has been receiving from many people at the hospital.

THE DEFENSE: The "excellent lawyer" part sounds delusional in and of itself.

THE WITNESS: Following that he began to tell me that one of the reasons he felt that he didn't deserve the treatment he had received was because of a feeling that he had that he was responsible for a variety of deaths.

Now, at this point I couldn't quite understand the content of what the defendant had said. I think it would have taken several more interviews, but I had the impression that he felt some of his words and some of his deeds were unacceptable to his family, and because of this they were feeling discouraged and negative about him, and that ultimately because of these feelings they would have to succumb in some fashion, but, as I say, I was quite puzzled about this aspect of the interview.

Following that he told me something about the accident that had taken place, and just prior to describing the accident he told me about his difficulties with the police, and he restricted it to the police in Precinct 8.

Now, he described this in a rather detailed fashion indicating to me that he felt the police were continually after him, that he was never safe, that anything that would occur in the area covered by Precinct 8 would be attributed to the defendant. He knew two officers in particular who were always reactive, always ready and willing to apprehend him independent of whether he had committed any crime.

He made one statement that I thought was very very interesting because he said to me, "They have two cars. There is a green Hudson and a gold Hudson, and I would know these cars anywhere. If you were to put the green Hudson in with one hundred green Hudsons exactly the same there is something about this policeman's car that I would sense and I would be able to recognize it even though they were all identical."

THE DEFENSE: What is the interpretation you attach to that statement, Doctor Levy?

THE WITNESS: This statement and the previous statement about the police made me feel that the defendant was describing a delusion he had about the police in that precinct.

Then he went on to indicate that he began to feel very uncomfortable, very tense, while he was in the car and didn't sense that there was anything he could do, and he began to speed and began to weave, and he had in mind finding a tree, and without any thought about his own safety he was eager to find that tree and then drive directly into it.

It was obvious from the way he described this that what must have taken place was a severe panic reaction, one in which he had virtually no control over his judgment or his impulses.

THE DEFENSE: Doctor Levy, did your tests in any way corroborate the conclusions that you drew from your clinical interview?

THE WITNESS: They did.

THE DEFENSE: Would you describe the tests, their results and your interpretations thereof?

THE WITNESS: The ink blot test—it is kind of unfortunate that it is called a test; it is not. It is a guided interview. The things that are used are ink blots and they are relatively standard and they are given to a subject or a patient, and the patient is asked to indicate what is seen on the ink blots.

The notion behind this is that the patient will see things on the ink blots and in the ink blots which are mirrored in the way he sees the world.

The court excluded a statement by the witness as to his opinion concerning the defendant's state of mind on June 9, 1960. In the words of the court: "He is not qualified to give a medical opinion as to whether he has schizophrenia or not; not in this court."

The line of questioning, therefore, followed a somewhat modified pattern, and I stressed the fact that I was calling for a *psychological* rather than any other kind of professional opinion from the witness.[17]

THE DEFENSE: Doctor Levy, would you explain to the court and the jury from your clinical interview and the test results that you obtained from this defendant the state of the defendant's personality as of the time of the examination in as much detail as you feel appropriate.

THE WITNESS: I think the most striking thing about the defendant's personality is the fact that it is covered over at the moment by a variety of psychological processes that keep it from coming into view. By analogy it is as though he were so terribly nervous that he couldn't express his essential self because there is something very very central in all of us that is ourselves and our

---

[17] Since the trial of this case, the Court of Appeals *has* explicitly ruled in Jenkins v. United States, 307 F.2d 637 (D.C. Cir. 1962), that appropriately qualified clinical psychologists were entitled to propound opinions as to the existence or nonexistence of a mental illness and that the exclusion of such opinions constituted error, warranting reversal.

uniqueness, and his essential uniqueness cannot come out because of the interfering processes. The major process that is interfering with the expression of himself is a very, very gross disorder of thinking, that is, he cannot reason logically, his ideas are peculiar to himself and probably not shared by anybody else. They are a result of a whole set of feelings, seething and very intense feelings that early in life should have been controlled, but now, because of some condition, he is unable to control, so that these feelings, very primitive feelings, of love and hate and aggression, and attempts to do violence, at least thoughts about this, violence to himself and to others, all of these things are seething and can't find expression easily because he hasn't gotten to the point in his life history to control these feelings.

In every instance this was apparent in the interview but made very dramatic in the ink blot test, where in every instance and in every ink blot he portrayed this kind of mixed up and confused idea of what the world is about.

THE DEFENSE: Now, do you have a psychological opinion, Doctor Levy, as to the length of time that this confused state of mind has existed within the defendant, [Walter X. Wilson]?

THE WITNESS: At the time that I worked with the defendant I had the opinion that this disease process, this psychological set of defects, was so intense, so severe, that it could have only developed over a long period of time.

. . .

THE DEFENSE: Is it fair to conclude then, Doctor Levy, it was in existence on June 9, 1960?

THE WITNESS: Yes.

THE DEFENSE: What would the effects of that state of mind have been on the mental and emotional processes of the defendant in specific terms?

THE WITNESS: For that period of time, at least, as he described it to me just prior to the accident, it would have robbed him of whatever reason and control he had, and would have enabled them, all of the impulses that he has been coping with throughout his life to find access and to motivate his behavior. At that time I think he was a very primitive person, and a person without a shred of judgment.[18]

The last psychologist to testify during that trial day was Mrs. Florence Kirby, who had administered the initial battery of psychological tests at the D.C. General Hospital in 1956 and had then administered a fresh battery at my request in 1961. Mrs. Kirby was an elderly lady with a sense of mission about the role of the psychologist in mental examinations. Her testimony was marked by a tone of fervent conviction and occasional indignation at attempts by the judge to disparage her testimony as inferior to that of a medical expert.

She reported that at the time of her first psychological examination of Walter, "[Walter] was showing the beginnings of a psychotic process or disorganization in his thinking. . . ." The balance of her testimony provided persuasive evidence of the fact that Walter had seriously deteriorated since that time.

When the court inquired with some degree of skepticism as to whether it was in her power to "give a Rorschach test alone and nothing else and reach a conclusion as to a man's mental condition," her "Yes, sir" provided answer, affirmation and protest at the same time.

Mrs. Kirby testified that she had spent a period of approximately three days testing Walter preliminary to the present trial in 1961. The forcefulness of her testimony and its easy acceptability to a lay audience, notwithstanding her

---

[18] My technique in this matter appears to have been noted with approval by a psychologist, observing the case for another NIH project who reported that I "was often able to get a reply by prefacing . . . my question with, 'your psychological opinion'—or, 'in your opinion as a psychologist.'" Scheflen, *supra* note 8.

occasional employment of technical terminology, can be highlighted by these samples from the transcript:

THE DEFENSE: Would you tell the court and the jury about the results that you obtained from the Rorschach test?

THE WITNESS: Well, the Rorschach test showed that this boy was in a much worse condition than he was on the previous date, that his fantasy life had increased tremendously, and that it had taken on a much more assaultive, much more gruesome type of content, and a much more hostile content, and a desire for vengeance, a retaliation against society or the world at large.

Also that his ego strength, or that part of the personality which had determined what is right or wrong by social standards, had decreased considerably; it was only about half [what] it was the previous time.

Also, that his control of his emotions, which is also indicated by the strength ego, had decreased tremendously. He was no longer able to control or to show foresight and determine the consequences of his conduct nearly as well—in fact, it was almost nil at this time as compared to the earlier test.

And much of his hostility was—practically all of his hostility was directed outward against other people.

At this time, this last test, there was no evidence on any tests that showed this boy had any feelings of conscience or regret; he was completely swallowed up with thoughts of hostility, of vengeance, of being captured, and escape, and electrocution, and all etcetera, associated with his present life.

THE DEFENSE: Mrs. Kirby, doesn't this make him identifiable as easily as a bad boy as a sick boy?

THE WITNESS: No, because of the difference in the strength of the ego from the two dates shows that this boy has lost control, voluntary control of his behavior. Also that his intellect has been so warped by his fantasy that he no longer sees things as real, as they actually are; he no longer interprets reality as it actually is; he is, in a sense, obsessed with these fantasies to a degree that he cannot stop them nor control them.

Succeeding questions were designed to pinpoint the existence of the mental illness in traditional terms.

THE DEFENSE: Do you believe this boy had control over his actions on June 9, 1960?
THE WITNESS: No. I think not.
THE DEFENSE: Do you believe, Mrs. Kirby, this boy had an understanding of the nature and quality of his actions on June 9, 1960?
THE WITNESS: I do not.[19]

Referring to the results of the Thematic Apperception Test, she pointed out that what was characteristic of the responses "was that each of these gave a short picture into this boy's home life, and it seemed to be permeated with erratic punishment, with rather unstable ethics, a great deal of severe punishment, and a great deal of rejection, and the actual pushing the boy out of the home, a play for dominance among the members of the home, and the boy feeling that he was unloved and not wanted and actually being pushed out of the door and out on the street, which, to him,

---

[19] It appeared ironic that the court which barred testimony by psychologists as to the existence of a schizophrenic mental state permitted psychologists to testify that the defendant lacked control over his actions and understanding of their nature and quality.

The employment of traditional terms designed to pinpoint defects in the volitional and cognitive capacities of the defendant was helpful to the insanity defense insofar as it was based upon psychotic symptomatology.

Adoption of the *Durham* rule had, at that time, not barred "all use of the older tests: testimony given in their terms" declared the Durham court, "might still be received if the expert witness feels able to give it . . . in resolving the ultimate issue 'whether the accused acted because of a mental disorder.' In aid of such a determination the court may permit the jury to consider whether or not the accused understood the nature of what he was doing. . . ." Douglas v. United States, 239 F.2d 52, 58 (D.C. Cir. 1956).

in the story is about as dramatic as walking a gang plank into the Atlantic Ocean."

There was no cross-examination of Mrs. Kirby.

Looking back upon the testimony of the three psychologists at this stage, it appeared that the value of this kind of testimony to the trial lawyer was in many ways as high as the best psychiatric testimony available.[20]

At the end of that trial day, I received a report from Dr. Charles Goshen, who had agreed to serve as a surrebuttal witness for the defense, that the defendant had, in his opinion, become mentally incompetent to participate in the proceedings as a result of the accumulating stress.

THE FOURTH DAY OF THE TRIAL

Upon the resumption of the trial, I informed the court of Dr. Goshen's findings at a bench conference. The court was further informed at that time by the prosecution that the government had doctors who would "look . . . [Walter] over" in aid of a judicial determination of competency to proceed in the case.

At the conclusion of this session, I requested both Dr.

---

[20] A psychologist observing the case for another N.I.H. project had these comments:

The psychologist's orientation in behavioral processes should lead him to think of mental illness in terms that are relatively clear and understandable. In addition, the specificity of his psychological tests offers a framework within which objective facts and observations can be offered. Also, the relative recency of psychology has forced those trained in this field to be prepared to defend the validity of their findings. . . .

. . . the psychologists in the case observed seemed to have done little previous testifying in the courtroom. Although questioned at great length by both the prosecuting attorney and the judge, they remained calm and definite in manner. This was probably due to their training in the description of behavior, the fact that their answers were concerning clinical psychological testing. The jury was very attentive to all of their testimony and one had the feeling that their testimony was accepted favorably.

Scheflen, *supra* note 8, at 331, 334.

Ryan and Dr. Salzman to make a further examination of the defendant as to his competency to stand trial.

Dr. Ryan telephoned me immediately after his examination to inform me of his opinion that the defendant was clearly incompetent to stand trial. He pointed to an unmistakable deterioration in the defendant's condition and added that he thought the defendant was suffering from the delusion that I had undergone a total change in appearance which suggested to him that he could no longer trust me and that I was part of the plot which had "rigged" the trial against him. In the opinion of Dr. Ryan, Walter was no longer capable of assisting counsel or participating in the proceedings. In the course of a later discussion, Dr. Ryan told me that he felt that something had occurred in the lawyer-client relationship in this case to help bring about this situation.

Dr. Salzman, in contrast, expressed no such feeling for the boy or the case. He telephoned at the conclusion of his examination to inquire as to what all the fuss was about, declared that he felt that the defendant was clearly competent to confer with counsel and assist in his own defense and quoted the defendant as saying that he regarded Dr. Salzman and me as the two best friends he had in the world.

THE FIFTH DAY OF THE TRIAL

A conference preceded the opening of the fifth day of the trial. The judge informed prosecuting and defense counsel that he had received letters from Doctors Platkin and Cushard of St. Elizabeths expressing their respective opinions after seeing the defendant, that the defendant was competent to proceed in his defense.[21]

---

[21] As was shown by the subsequent hospital records of St. Elizabeths, obtained at a later date, the interview which led Drs. Platkin and Cushard to pronounce Walter X. Wilson competent to stand trial produced evidence that Walter X. Wilson expressed the delusion "that he had killed four boys, two of whom he knew, in Rock Creek Park and buried their bodies."

He further informed both counsel that he had received a letter from Dr. Ryan to the contrary and he added that he just did not know what to make of so sharp a conflict of opinion among reputable professional men. He inquired whether any further evidence was available upon the subject.

I informed the judge and prosecuting counsel that Dr. Goshen was available to testify as to the defendant's lack of competency at this time, adding that Dr. Salzman had informed me that defendant was, in his opinion, competent.

Proceedings thereupon were resumed in open court. The court heard evidence outside the hearing of the jury. Dr. Goshen testified that in his opinion the defendant was at that stage "unable to understand the nature of the proceedings . . . and unable to rationally participate in his own defense." He added that "the trial itself as accompanied by incarceration in the jail . . . constitutes a great stress on him to the point where when I saw him . . . he was suicidal at that time."

The court thereupon declared:

> It has been agreed that the court should consider the report of Doctor Cushard, Doctor Platkin, Doctor Ryan, and the testimony of Doctor Goshen.
>
> Doctor Cushard has reported that he concludes that [Walter X. Wilson] is mentally competent to stand trial and understand the nature of the proceedings against him, and properly assist counsel in his own defense.
>
> Doctor Platkin expresses an opinion that [Walter X. Wilson] is competent to stand trial and understand the nature of the proceedings against him, and properly assist counsel in his own defense.
>
> Doctor Goshen has testified in his opinion he is not competent to stand trial, and Doctor Ryan reports that at the present time Mr. [Wilson] appears to be in a state of acute psychotic turmoil. This is dated March 31, 1961. And it is possible that he may erupt in violent behavior in court. He feels convinced that his lawyer has undergone a total change in appearance which suggests to him that he can no longer trust his attorney because he too is in a plot against him. He views the jury as constantly changing in makeup from almost all men to almost all women, or almost all colored to almost all white. He is also presently disoriented as to time whereas he was correctly oriented a week ago.

Throughout the examination he showed considerably more confusion and disorder in logical thinking than he did [two weeks ago]. It is thus my opinion that Mr. [Wilson] is not now competent to stand trial.

The picture presents itself as two psychiatrists expressing an opinion that he is competent to stand trial, and two psychiatrists expressing an opinion that he is not capable to stand trial. The condition of the record is such that I hold that he is not capable of standing trial and I will declare a mistrial.

Counsel for the government will prepare the proper order.

He will be committed to St. Elizabeths.

POST TRIAL EVENTS

Some time after Walter's commitment for a ninety-day period to St. Elizabeths Hospital, the defense filed a motion for the appointment at government expense, of Doctors Schultz, Ryan and Goshen for further mental examination to bring their findings up to date.

As I set forth the facts underlying the motion, beginning with the initial diagnosis of mental illness in 1956 and the subsequent rejection of that diagnosis and discharge of the boy by St. Elizabeths Hospital in the same year, the Judge, hearing the motion, observed:

> This is certainly a sad commentary on our handling of these psychiatric cases, where these psychiatrists are debating among themselves and as a result a man of this nature can go out and kill four innocent people. It isn't the first time it's happened. I am afraid it isn't going to be the last. It is, I think, one of the greatest blots on our system of justice that I know of. . . .

Though opposed by the government, the motion was granted.

When I visited Walter at St. Elizabeths Hospital, I requested him to keep a chart showing specifically what doctor had seen him and for what length of time.

On my next visit, Walter informed me that his chart had been taken from him by one of the attendants who had told him that if he persisted in such activities he would be asking for trouble. I asked Walter to persist nonetheless. Toward the end of the ninety-day period, Walter's chart, which he had managed to keep this time, showed approximately five interviews with medical staff members of the hospital.

Significantly, at the conclusion of the ninety-day period of observation, St. Elizabeths Hospital reported that the patient was mentally ill although competent to stand trial. The hospital was unable to express an opinion as to the relationship of the "crime" to the mental disorder. The finding of a schizophrenic mental disorder was supported by the hospital records.[22]

[22] ". . . [Walter X. Wilson] was readmitted to Saint Elizabeths Hospital April 3, 1961, by order of the United States District Court for the District of Columbia for a period of not to exceed 90 days. . . . Opinions are requested as to the patient's present mental condition, mental competency for trial, mental condition on or about June 9, 1960 and causal connection between the mental disease or defect if present and the alleged criminal act: Manslaughter. . . .

The patient's account of the night of the alleged offense is essentially the same as that given in the Medical Staff Conference dated February 15, 1961, during the patient's second admission to the hospital and will therefore not be repeated here. The patient is considerably more emotionally disturbed now than during conference of February 15, 1961. Asked how he feels, the patient says, 'scared and don't know what I'm scared of.' He says that he sees no hope at all for the future. He says that half the people in Washington are against him and the [Wilson] family and would not even give them public assistance, as a result of which his mother had to go out and work instead of staying at home. Questioned closely as to whether he really believes that half the people in Washington are against him and his family he changes the statement and says that all the people in Washington are against them. He says that nobody in the world likes him and that he does not like anyone and does not get along with anyone. He has no desire to have anything to do with anyone either here in the hospital or outside. He says that while driving the car he wanted to kill himself and is sorry that he didn't. He says that there is no reason for him to continue living. It is the impression of several members of the conference that this patient's contact with reality is quite tenuous and has been so particularly at certain times. He is correctly oriented and his memory shows no significant impairment. He does not express delusions, hallucinations or other psychotic content. I should like to note at this time, however, that Dr. Platkin and the writer [Dr, Cushard] examined this patient at the D.C. Jail, on a court order, between his second and third admissions to this hospital and at that time he expressed the opinion that he had killed four boys, two

(Footnote continued on next page.)

Dr. Platkin appeared to be the sole dissenter from this viewpoint. His assertion continued to be that the boy was free of all manner of mental disorder.

---

of whom he knew, in Rock Creek Park and buried their bodies. He said that he was so convinced that he had done this that he went back to find the graves and was unable to do so. For some time during that examination he insisted that this had actually happened, but finally admitted that it might be an illusion. Questioned about this today he again states that it was an illusion. He says that he hates everyone so that if he continues to live he will hurt and kill people. During parts of the examination the patient seems more absorbed in his own thoughts than in what is going on in the conference, but he does not become completely detached from reality.

Psychological testing showed the patient to have a full scale I.Q. of 77, verbal I.Q. of 82, and performance I.Q. of 73, and his probable *maximum* was estimated as at least average. He attained the full scale. I.Q. of 77 on the Wechsler adult intelligence scale as compared with an I.Q. of 90 on the Stanford-Binet, when he was in the hospital in 1956. The psychological test results reflected conflict, extreme anxiety and panic over impulses for which the patient has inadequate controls. Emotions are lived out directly and immediately. The fear of loss of control is too great to be tolerated for long and under stress may be projected on the environment. So much inner energy is used in the struggle for mastery that very little is left for relating to the environment. Language is functional and at times marked by looseness of associations and autistic coloring. Such a person can eventually move into paranoid schizoprenia.

During his second admission to the hospital this patient was diagnosed as without mental disorder because it was not believed that he deviated sufficiently from normal to warrant a diagnosis of mental disorder. It is the consensus of opinion at this time in view of the patient's condition and subsequent examinations that he is so disturbed that he does suffer from a mental disorder. It is the consensus of opinion that simple schizophrenia is probably the most accurate diagnosis which can be made, although not entirely satisfactorily. It is also the consensus of opinion that the patient was suffering from mental disorder on June 9, 1960, but we are unable to arrive at a firm opinion as to whether or not there was causal connection between the alleged criminal act and the mental illness.

Diagnosis: 22.0 Schizophrenic Reaction Simple Type.

Condition on Discharge: Unimproved

Recommendations: In our opinion:
1. He is mentally competent for trial.
2. He is suffering from a mental disorder and was in probability suffering from a mental disorder on or about June 9, 1960. We are unable to arrive at a valid opinion as to whether the criminal acts if committed by him were the products of a mental disorder."

Doctors Ryan and Goshen, who had checked upon their patient at St. Elizabeths Hospital pursuant to court order toward the end of the ninety-day period, agreed that he was then again competent to stand trial although clearly schizophrenic.

I furnished the St. Elizabeths photostats to the United States Attorney's office, and suggested that this was a case in which the government might not wish to contest the insanity defense.

My opposite number in the United States Attorney's Office called me to say that the matter was being taken under advisement. When I discussed it in his office a day afterwards, he informed me that Dr. Platkin strongly dissented from the present hospital diagnosis of mental disorder and maintained that the defendant was, and had been, without mental disorder at all critical periods under consideration. I asked as to whether he was aware of the fact that Dr. Platkin had just failed the examinations conducted by the American Board of Psychiatry and Neurology. He replied that he was and inquired if I planned to use this information upon cross-examination of Dr. Platkin. My reply, as far as I can recall, was something like: "What would you do if you were in my position?"

I received a telephone call from the United States Attorney's Office the next morning and was informed that the government had decided not to contest the insanity defense.

THE SECOND TRIAL

The second trial was, of course, anticlimactic. A jury was waived. The court received in evidence the transcript of testimony of the first trial. It also heard the testimony of Dr. Charles Goshen, who had reexamined the boy during his second sojourn at the hospital. There was no cross-examination. There were no opposing witnesses.

The court entered a judgment of acquittal by reason of insanity and committed Walter to St. Elizabeths Hospital until such time as he could be certified as recovered and no longer dangerous to himself or others.

The proceedings in their entirety did not consume more than twenty minutes.

CONCLUSION

The outcome of the case hinged plainly and dramatically upon availability of necessary funds to secure the various examinations and reexaminations which have been described. "Therefore put money in thy purse."

It is clear in this light that if the war on poverty is to be extended into the domain of criminal defense, the skirmish of the *Wilson* case highlights the need for a greater investment in financial and human resources—particularly in the field of psychiatric and psychological expertise—than it has received to date. To bring about a reevaluation of a St. Elizabeths diagnosis requires the use of psychiatric experts whose services must be purchased.

It is also similarly clear that selection of psychiatrists for the defense can be hazardous.

CHAPTER VII

HERESY IN THE COURTROOM: THE DEFENSE OF A DRUG ADDICT AS MENTALLY ILL

The treatment of the drug addict is marked by what is perhaps the uttermost in savagery encountered in American legal practice. Unlike the murderer or traitor who, in theory at least, may secure his freedom after a period of expiation, the confirmed drug addict is subject to mandatory sentences running into decades and indeed life without any possibility of probation or parole.[1]

Reliance upon the insanity defense in such a case appears to be the only legally countenanced escape from this draconian severity.

He who would assert such a defense for the addict must however count on hostility discoverable in a courtroom only in rare cases of treason, murder and sedition.

The case of *United States v. Rivers*[2] is a case in point.

A NARCOTICS VIOLATOR SEEKS ASSISTANCE

On September 15, 1961, Narcotics Officers executing a search warrant entered a shabbily furnished room on the third floor of a building located at 515—7th Street, Southeast, in the City of Washington, D.C. where they encountered

---

[1] For documentation, *see* Appendix III.

[2] A pseudonym has been used in this case, therefore no attempt is made to support any colloquies by reference to the actual transcript.

James Rivers lying on his bed in his underwear. His wife, fully dressed, was sitting beside him.

When they asked James Rivers whether he had any narcotics in the room, he nodded affirmance, pointing toward the top right-hand dressing-table drawer.

One of the narcotics officers opened the drawer and took from it a leather case containing a cream colored envelope with eighty-one gelatin capsules.

The case also contained an eye dropper, syringes and some hypodermic needles.

James Rivers was arrested and taken to police headquarters for interrogation where he signed an "addict form" in the presence of narcotics officers.

He subsequently asserted that he was by that time in the throes of withdrawal symptoms for which he received no treatment at police headquarters.

A two-count indictment was returned against him by a Grand Jury on January 15, 1962 charging violation of the federal narcotics law[3]—specifically the concealment and possession of contraband drugs. If convicted, he faced a minimum sentence of ten years imprisonment on each count without any possibility of parole as a second narcotics offender.

The *Rivers* case had originally been assigned to one of the Georgetown University legal interns.

The intern, Mr. Kenneth Schroeder, duly moved for mental examination of his client at St. Elizabeths Hospital. St. Elizabeths Hospital had by that time transmitted its routine certification to the court, asserting that:

> . . . . As a result of our examinations and observation, it is our opinion that Mr. [James Rivers] . . . is mentally competent

---

[3] Violation: 26 U.S.C. 4704 (a); 21 U.S.C. 174 (Possession of narcotic drugs; facilitation of concealment and sale of narcotic drugs, knowing same to have been imported contrary to law.) [The sections have since been respectively renumbered as 21 U.S.C. 951 and 21 U.S.C. 951-6 without significant change in penalties.]

to understand the nature of the proceedings against him and to consult properly with counsel in his own defense. We find no evidence of mental disease existing at the present time nor on or about December 15, 1961. He is not suffering from mental deficiency.

Mr. Schroeder asked me to accept the case as trial counsel. His reasons were twofold. The Georgetown Legal Internship Program was terminating its operations at the conclusion of the academic year 1961-62 for the summer recess but, perhaps more importantly, Mr. Schroeder had, as he subsequently expressed it, his own opinion concerning the value of the St. Elizabeths diagnostic work-up. He also believed that since the Project on Law and Psychiatry had the money and resources to afford psychiatric assistance to his client, he was duty bound by the Canons of Ethics to further the cause of his client by turning to me when he did.

A DEFENSE LAWYER SEEKS PSYCHIATRISTS IN AID OF A HANDICAPPED CLIENT

Although well financed to provide Mr. Rivers with precisely the psychiatric assistance which he needed, I found it extremely difficult to secure psychiatric witnesses for his case.

While an N.I.H. grant specifically authorizing the expenditure of funds for psychiatric testimony had been in effect for well over a year, I had not, until this case, succeeded in obtaining a rotating panel of psychiatrists from the Washington School of Psychiatry.

Outside of two psychiatrists who were generally available, I had found it impossible to recruit a group of professionals which was available for courtroom testimony. A typical experience would be that of telephoning thirty to forty psychiatrists and obtaining one. By the summer of 1962, however, a psychiatric committee of the Washington School of

Psychiatry had succeeded in securing a group of volunteers which was to be made available on the basis of mechanical rotation. Even then, however, the availability of psychiatric experts seemed haphazard.

Several weeks before the Rivers trial only Dr. George W. Sprehn had explicitly pledged his support in the examination and evaluation of the patient.

The doctors who were finally made available for the defendant's case primarily through the Committee of the Washington School of Psychiatry, were Doctors George Warren Sprehn and William Clotworthy. Both became members of what was subsequently known among court officials and the representatives of the local press as "the Arens stable of psychiatrists."

A third psychiatrist, whom I succeeded in contacting on my own and who, up to that point at least, had not incurred the stigma of a member of the "stable," was Dr. Wilbur Hamman of St. Elizabeths Hospital.

I had also contacted a former President of the American Psychiatric Association. He had spoken volubly about the psychiatric irresponsibility of labeling a chronic narcotics addict as anything but mentally ill and had expressed his indignation at what he conceived to be the practices of St. Elizabeths Hospital in this matter. Accordingly, I asked one of my assistants to serve him with a subpoena at his office. Some time that afternoon, I received a telephone call from this physician. Using a wide range of four letter expletives, he informed me in what appeared to be a highly agitated state that my behavior was outrageous. He announced that he would not testify in the case and that he would rather leave town than answer the subpoena, and he added that any lawyer concerned with his professional future would turn and run as fast as his legs could carry him at the sight of any narcotics case. He seemed only mildly mollified when I informed him that I would not compel his appearance, and continued a soliloquy at some length along his earlier lines.

Dr. Sprehn was a practicing psychiatrist and psychoanalyst, and Director of the Community Psychiatric Clinic in Bethesda, Maryland. He was readily available for conferences and referred to any prisoner whom he examined as his "patient." He examined James Rivers twice at the D.C. Jail prior to the trial and he also interviewed his wife and foster father.

Dr. Clotworthy was one of the younger psychoanalysts in town. He was also a member of the Mental Health Commission. As his doubts about his participation remained unresolved for some time, I did not succeed in meeting with him until the eve of the trial. When I encountered him by accident at the D.C. Jail, I showed him Dr. Sprehn's preliminary report as well as a report of the Social Welfare Department.

My only further contacts with him consisted of a few telephone conversations. Beyond this he was unavailable to the defense.

Dr. Clotworthy saw James Rivers on but one occasion preliminary to the trial.

Outside the realm of the Washington School panel of rotating psychiatrists, Dr. Wilbur Hamman, who joined the defense, was one of the younger staff members of the maximum security division of St. Elizabeths Hospital. He had participated at a St. Elizabeths staff conference on James Rivers.[4]

He had committed himself in an earlier case[5] to the view that a narcotics addict was mentally ill. He had done so

---

[4] The United States Attorney's office appeared to reflect the view that the younger staff members at St. Elizabeths Hospital are "liberal" and insufficiently "skeptical" in the evaluation of the problem of criminal responsibility. *See* Acheson, *McDonald v. United States; The Durham Rule Redefined*, 51 GEO. L. J. 580, 588 (1963).

[5] United States v. Wallace H. Carroll, Crim. No. 383-62. Official Transcript—Vol. 1, Testimony of Dr. Leonard J. Hantsoo, Dr. John Porter Fort, Dr. Wilbur A. Hamman, Dr. Lawrence Kolb, June 21, 22 and 25, 1962, pp. 56 to 88.

both upon the basis of a hypothetical question[6] as well as

---

[6] The hypothetical question addressed to him on that occasion had read as follows:

MR. McDONALD: Now, Doctor, I am going to ask you to assume the following facts:

"A man is twenty-eight years of age, of the Negro race, his parents separated when he was nine years old. His father left town at that time, and the man has never seen his father since.

The man left school after the tenth grade. In the same year the house he was living in was repossessed. He thus was separated from his mother, and lived with friends.

He joined the Navy approximately a year later. He states that he always felt unloved by his parents, and he feels, he states, that the world is against him. This feeling, according to him, becomes intensified when he's in crowds, where he becomes quite tense and begins to perspire and sweat exceedingly.

In 1951, he began using drugs in Japan while in the Navy. Thereafter he became addicted to them.

While using drugs, he states that he feels much better; his tension is lessened, and he has a sense of well-being.

After getting out of the Navy, he worked for the Norfolk Naval Base and attempted to kick this drug habit. After approximately eleven months, he quit to go live in Jacksonville, Florida. He did not succeed in kicking his drug habit.

After returning to Jacksonville, Florida, he attempted to again kick his drug habit. During this period of time while he was attempting to kick his drug habit, he would go through sicknesses.

He worked five months as a cook trainee, and was fired. And then worked about three more months in the Federal Building as a janitor, and lost his job. He was unemployed the remainder of this time there in Florida.

During this time he used, among other drugs, cocaine, and while under the influence, he had dreams of being trapped in a hole and of snakes.

In 1959 he came to live in Washington, in the Washington area, and again attempted to kick his drug habit. During this time he would substitute liquor for the drugs he was not getting.

He began to work at a hotel as a porter and bellhop, and at first did his work to the satisfaction of his employer. While working at the hotel over the next twenty months, he attempted on at least two occasions to kick his drug habit without success.

Eventually his employer saw that his work was not being done in a satisfactory manner, that on work breaks he would return in a woozy condition and appear doped up. This man's attitude finally led to his having argumentative outbursts with guests, and finally led to his being fired in May of 1961—excuse me—strike that—of his being fired in the spring of 1961.

His landlord, his employers and employees have described him as being exceptionally moody, with periods of extreme talkativeness changing to

(Footnote continued on next page.)

upon psychiatric examination. It was obvious that in taking this stand, he was acting contrary to what appeared to be the dominant policy, set by the senior staff members of the maximum security division of St. Elizabeths Hospital.[7]

As a member of the St. Elizabeths staff he felt disqualified from pretrial planning with defense counsel and restricted himself to a discussion of the "mental status" of James Rivers over the telephone.

I met James Rivers in the District jail for the usual first interview. He was a thirty-seven year old Negro from an obviously lower income background, wore an artificial leg and moved about with difficulty. He appeared despondent in the extreme. His handshake was limp. His eyes were often fixed upon the floor and his tone was one of almost overwhelming sadness. He at no time evaded answering any of my questions, yet he at no time volunteered an answer which might have evoked sympathy.

After several personal interviews, he appeared to gain confidence that he would receive significant legal support. He talked more freely and his handshake became firm. Beyond this, there appeared to be no change in his demeanor.

---

periods of quietness and sullenness. He was also attracted to the Muslim religion during this period of time.

During the period from January 1st to the end of March, March 28th of this year, 1962, he was taking approximately thirty-five to fifty capsules of heroin each day.

After being fired from his hotel job, in order to support this narcotic habit, he began to sell a sufficient amount of drugs to do this. In addition, he supplemented this heroin dosage over the last few months, from January to March, 1962, by drinking approximately one to two pints of wine per day.

Upon his arrest on March 28th, his drug supply was cut off. He went through a period of sickness. His illness was characterized by weird dreams and by dry heaves, which included the spitting of blood. A physical examination by jail doctors showed scars on his arms, old and recent scars on his arms, legs, feet, cubital regions." *Id.,* 58-61.

[7] *See* United States v. Wallace Carroll, Crim. No. 383-62 Official Transcript Vol. I, Testimony of Dr. Leonard J. Hantsoo, Dr. John Porter Fort, Dr. Willbur A. Hamman, Dr. Lawrence Kolb, June 21, 22 and 25, 1962, *passim.*

Maximal disclosure by him was made not to me but to psychiatrists retained for the defense, although it is worth noting in this connection that the psychiatrists entered the case at a time when James Rivers' belief that he was about to be helped was at its height.

James Rivers himself claimed never to have been interviewed in any private session by any staff member of St. Elizabeths Hospital except for a combined physical examination and interview to which he was subjected on admission, and for some psychological testing.

The nature of James Rivers' impoverished background is perhaps best set forth in a letter addressed to me by the Department of Public Welfare of the District of Columbia which provided the following facts:

> ... [He] was first known to the Department of Public Welfare on 1-12-28 after he was abandoned by his mother in the home of an unrelated caretaker. The persons named as parents appeared in court, but the man denied paternity, and denied that the woman who claimed to be the mother was the natural mother. His denial of her claim to maternity was supported by her relatives. The so-called mother disappeared for several years, and reappeared when ... [he] was sixteen years old, but failed to convince either agency or ... [James] of her relationship. ... [James] felt, however, that the woman knew the whereabouts of his mother. She dropped out of the picture in 1945 when ... [his] leg was amputated saying that she hoped that he would be dead the next time she heard from him.

Doctors Sprehn and Clotworthy both noted what they regarded as the man's earnestness and ability to "stir someone's interest in him."

Dr. Sprehn diagnosed his patient as suffering from a neurotic depressive reaction. Dr. Clotworthy diagnosed him as a sociopathic personality with depressive features. Significantly after making this diagnosis in his report, Dr. Clotworthy declared:

> Such is the nature of the difficulty in categorizing persons that to me almost as good a case could be made for the diagnosis of neurotic depressive reaction with drug addiction and antisocial behavior.

Dr. Sprehn in turn expressed the view that his diagnosis was in no way inconsistent with that of Dr. Clotworthy's.

Dr. Hamman lacked the data for as comprehensive a report on James Rivers as was furnished by Doctors Sprehn and Clotworthy. He expressed the view that Rivers' pattern of maladjustment was most probably consistent with that of an "inadequate personality," but went on to say that this diagnostic impression was in no way inconsistent with the diagnosis furnished by Doctors Sprehn and Clotworthy.

I did not feel that I could produce anything beyond this degree of agreement in the assessment of the defendant's mental state by his experts. Nor did I feel that a greater degree of synchronization of diagnostic views was necessary, as all three experts appeared to share essentially the same general perspective in the description of James Rivers' condition. I therefore did not press for agreement upon an identical diagnostic verbal label by our medical witnesses.

What concerned me more than the apparent rather than the real split on diagnoses was the fact that my medical witnesses would face the claim by St. Elizabeths physicians that the St. Elizabeths view was entitled to greater weight insofar as it was based on ninety days' intensive studies and observation. I proposed to attack this problem through the cross-examination of St. Elizabeths witnesses as to the inadequacy of existing hospital facilities for reliable diagnostic work. St. Elizabeths was committed to the view that mentally and emotionally healthy drug addicts were indeed discoverable, at least upon their premises. I sought, as I had done in the *Wilson* case, the services of an independent psychiatrist, willing to engage in an evaluation of the adequacy of the diagnostic work-up performed by the St. Elizabeths staff as reflected by the hospital record. Through the rotating panel established by the Washington School of Psychiatry, I secured the services of Dr. Randolf Frank, a former psychiatric staff member of the Federal Narcotics Hospital at Lexington. Dr. Frank agreed to review James Rivers' hospital records. These I had obtained by subpoena. He informed me that he would not have the time to examine the defendant.

When I presented the hospital records to Dr. Frank at a weekend meeting with him at a colleague's home, he exclaimed, after glancing at them briefly:

"Why, they haven't even run the most elementary tests."

After further study of the records, he asserted that it appeared plain to him that essential neurological procedures designed to rule out brain damage, had been omitted in the hospital study of the defendant. He further informed me that such data as appeared in the record pointed to the presence of a mental disease. As expressed by Dr. Frank in a final evaluation of the record some two months after trial, "the St. Elizabeths' diagnostic work-up was grossly incomplete, inconsistent and inadequate."[8]

As the trial date approached I became puzzled by a sudden change in the attitude of the jail officials toward me and my staff. Unaccountably, for example, a student assistant whom I had asked to check with James Rivers on details of his testimony on the eve of trial was denied admission to the District Jail. I myself was kept waiting beyond the usual period on visits to my client during the last days preceding the commencement of the trial itself.

THE FIRST DAY OF THE TRIAL, JULY 3, 1962

A senior member of the United States Attorney's office represented the government.

My first act in court consisted of asking the judge's permission to have a law student, who was assisting me, seated at the counsel table. Permission to do this was granted with what appeared to be obvious reluctance on the judge's part. The jurors, selected without exhaustion of the

---

[8] Letter to Counsel, dated August 9, 1962.

peremptory challenges available to both counsel, were a bookkeeper, a statistician, an engineer, an accountant, a stamp examiner, two housewives, an archivist, a "consultant," an administrative officer, a cartographer and a statistical clerk. Two alternate jurors were selected without challenge. One was listed as a printer, the other as retired.

I confess to having paid insufficient attention to the impact of the alternate jurors upon the basic atmosphere of jury deliberation and hence had not interposed a challenge to alternate juror No. 2 who had listed himself as retired. I would have been inclined to challenge him if he had been selected as a regular juror, upon the basis of his years and an apparent air of rigidity of outlook.

That particular alternate juror sat through the entire trial in the jury box, never ceasing to smile with obvious incredulity and amazement at what must have struck him as the "crazy" defense of insanity for a drug addict.

The usual opening for the prosecution was followed by the opening for the defense.

This was interrupted by the court when I stated that the defendant had never learned to read and write because he "was too full of fears in his early years." I was told that I was argumentative.

The prosecution's case in chief was then established by two narcotics officers and a chemist.

I attempted to establish upon cross-examination that James Rivers possessed the equipment characteristic of a drug addict. This evidence was elicited with considerable difficulty. Action by the court made it inevitable that it was complemented by the witness' opinion that the equipment in question was also characteristic of that of a peddler.

This is how the cross-examination was shaped under the circumstances:

THE DEFENSE: Now, Officer Paul, you are an experienced
    member of the Narcotics Squad of the Metropolitan
    Police Department. Would it be fair to say, the exhibits

which you have identified, are characteristic of the equipment of narcotic addicts that you have dealt with in the course of your experience?

THE PROSECUTION: If Your Honor please, I must object.

THE COURT: Characteristic of an addict, sir?

THE DEFENSE: Of the equipment carried by an addict.

THE PROSECUTION: I must object to the form of the question. Characteristic of an addict, sir.

THE COURT: Reframe it, Mr. Arens.

THE DEFENSE: I will withdraw it. May we approach the bench?

THE COURT: Yes, sir.

(BENCH CONFERENCE.)

THE DEFENSE: I would like the witness' opinion as an expert, if it is the practice of addicts to carry such items with an eye to letting the jury know this defendant was such an addict.

THE COURT: Do you want to admit he was an addict?

THE DEFENSE: Yes.

THE COURT: As a matter of fact, I think you are going to get more but you can ask it if you want to. You may get that it is also equipment of a peddler. Do you want that?

THE DEFENSE: Yes, Your Honor, I do.

(END OF BENCH CONFERENCE)

THE DEFENSE: Officer Paul, would the items you identified for the Government be typical, in your opinion, of equipment carried by narcotic addicts?

THE WITNESS: I would not state for all addicts, no, sir. Some were and some were not.

THE DEFENSE: Which were and which were not?

THE WITNESS: I would say a person who is a narcotic addict, they usually have the addict paraphernalia which consists of your syringes, cookers and hypodermic needles.

THE DEFENSE: And the defendant had all of these?
THE WITNESS: Yes, sir, these he had.
THE DEFENSE: Thank you, Officer Paul. I have no further questions.
THE WITNESS: May I—
THE COURT: Yes, you may finish.
THE WITNESS: Now, he also had along with that, he had a large quantity of capsules which had traces. I usually find these in places where the person is selling narcotics, a narcotic peddler.

I had no recollection that this prosecution witness had lowered his voice and was startled to hear the prosecutor exclaim:

I did not hear that.

The answer was, of course, a reaffirmation of the theme of drug-peddling:

Where a person is selling drugs. Also he had here a box containing empty gelatin capsules. These I usually find also where a person is selling narcotic drugs.
Also, the strainer here, I always find this in places where a person is selling narcotic drugs, something similiar to this and this would be indicative of a peddler rather than a user, just a plain addict.

Redirect examination is caught in this excerpt from the transcript.

THE DEFENSE: The items *in toto* represent items carried by an addict and a peddler, is that correct?
THE WITNESS: I would say that, yes.
THE DEFENSE: Thank you very much.
THE COURT: All right, you may step down.

The second narcotics officer admitted that the defendant was a narcotic addict because of needle marks which he had displayed to him. He denied that the defendant had experienced any withdrawal symptoms in his presence, and further asserted that the defendant had read an "Addict Form" and that he therefore concluded that he was not illiterate.

Only one other witness was at that stage expected to be called to conclude the Government's case in chief.

The brevity of the Government's case in chief necessitated the immediate alerting of defense psychiatrists to be on call to answer an immediate summons to appear in court.

Accordingly, I passed messages to a student assistant, sitting at the counsel table, that various doctors were to be telephoned and informed as to the anticipated time of their testimony.

Dr. Sprehn, who had made arrangements to conduct a further psychiatric interview at the jail on the evening of July 3 was thus to be informed, according to the instructions I had scribbled on one of the messages passed to the student assistant, that he was to make a further check on the literacy of the defendant—in the light of the testimony of one of the narcotics officers that he had considered the defendant literate.

These messages were taken by the student assistant and handed to a Mrs. Janet Pomeranz, a social scientist connected with the project and seated in one of the front rows of the spectators' seats. Mrs. Pomeranz would, upon receipt of these messages, leave the courtroom and put through the necessary telephone calls.

All of this took place in the full view of the court and prosecution.

Dr. Sprehn, waiting in the witness room to be called to testify, reported that the efforts made by the defense counsel and his staff to minimize his loss of time had resulted in charges of "collusion" between the witnesses and counsel's staff by members of the Marshal's office.

I attempted at that stage to accept a suggestion made by a member of the prosecutor's staff that a marshal be utilized to check upon the presence of witnesses who had arrived. Significantly, however, the marshal and his assistants were unable or unwilling on all but one occasion to leave their posts within the courtroom to comply with a request essential to the orderly presentation of the defense. Accordingly, my assistants had to be requested once again to leave the courtroom to make certain that the witnesses were available. I sought to prevent any further charge of collusion by approaching the bench in the midst of an examination of a witness by the government to inform the court that a law student, assisting me in the case, was leaving the courtroom to notify an expert witness that he could be expected to be called in short order. The court responded with absolute silence.

The third prosecution witness was a government chemist who testified to the narcotic content of forty-three capsules seized in the defendant's apartment.

There was no cross-examination.

The government rested.

I moved for a judgment of acquittal by reason of insanity on the ground that the government's case in chief had produced evidence of narcotics addiction which was "some evidence of insanity" undisputed by any other evidence in the field. The motion was denied.

Both narcotics officers, upon leaving the stand, seated themselves conspicuously in a front row of the spectators' seats in the courtroom. They retained that position until close to the end of the trial. They exchanged whispered confidences with other individuals who presumably were colleagues. Throughout much of the testimony, a marked smile of incredulity never left them. This appeared particularly pronounced as the first witness for the defense—the defendant himself—took the stand, but it did not seem to leave them in the presence of the expert witnesses. Sometimes their facial features alternated between smile and consternation.[9] They were joined by other members of their staff.

James Rivers had slumped over the counsel table throughout most of the prosecution testimony.

When called upon to take the stand as the first witness for the defense, he rose and limped painfully to the witness stand.

His direct examination was reflected as follows in the trial transcript:

THE DEFENSE: Mr. . . . [Rivers] would you state your full name to the court and the Jury?
THE WITNESS: . . . [James Rivers]
THE DEFENSE: You are the defendant in this case?
THE WITNESS: Yes, sir.
THE DEFENSE: . . . Are you now or have you ever been a drug addict?
THE WITNESS: I am a drug addict.
THE DEFENSE: Have you ever been hospitalized for drug addiction?
THE WITNESS: Yes, sir, I have.
THE DEFENSE: When was that, sir? . . .
THE WITNESS: I was hospitalized twice. Once in Lexington and once in D.C. General Hospital.
THE DEFENSE: How much time did you spend in those two hospitals?
THE WITNESS: I was in Lexington, Kentucky, in 1945—1954 and I stayed in Lexington about eight months. I didn't

---

[9] I believed that the atmosphere of the trial was already too charged with tension for me to venture on what seemed at that stage a peripheral issue and one likely to call for the resolution of a question of fact by an antagonized judge. Accordingly, I did not make the matter of facial demonstration a matter of record.

It is not irrelevant to note that a judge presiding over another case, did not hesitate to bar considerably milder manifestations of facial incredulity upon hearing of government psychiatrists *sua sponte*.

See United States v. Ray, Crim. No. 250-61, Official Transcript of Testimony of Dr. Platkin and Dr. Owens, May 23, 1962.

continue my cure there and I was in D.C. General for a week and then didn't continue my cure there.
THE DEFENSE: When was that?
THE WITNESS: That was in 1960.
THE DEFENSE: ... When did you start taking narcotics?
THE WITNESS: I started taking narcotics back in 1945.
THE DEFENSE: What kind of narcotics were you taking at that time?
THE WITNESS: I was taking heroin.
THE DEFENSE: And did you become addicted?
THE WITNESS: Yes, sir, I did.
THE DEFENSE: Now what does being addicted mean to you?
THE WITNESS: Well, addicted means to me as if you were to get your meals and things like that, the same as I would like drugs. You have to have your meals and I have to have drugs.
THE DEFENSE: What happens to you if you don't have the drugs?
THE WITNESS: Well, I become—get sick, pains in my stomach, my eyes begin to run and I get a different type of sickness. It is hard to describe. It is miserable to you. I just get real sick inside.
THE DEFENSE: Now, when you first started taking heroin, how much did you take?
THE WITNESS: When I first started, I started one to two pills a day.
THE DEFENSE: And did you progressively increase this dose?
THE WITNESS: As I went along, yes, sir. As I come to be addicted to the drug, I didn't feel as though I felt when I first taken them so—
THE COURT: Did you increase the—
THE WITNESS: Yes, sir.
THE DEFENSE: How many pills or capsules were you taking at or near the time of your arrest?
THE WITNESS: I was taking ten to fifteen. As much as I could get my hands on.
THE DEFENSE: Ten to fifteen capsules a day?

The Witness: Yes, sir.
The Defense: ... Do you remember your parents?
The Witness: No, sir.
The Defense: Do you remember anyone who looked after you in your childhood?
The Witness: Well, after I was from, say, about eight years old, I remember—start remembering people, my foster mother, Mrs. Hawkins.
The Defense: Do you remember any foster parents before Mrs. Hawkins?
The Witness: I remember I used to live in northeast Washington and a lady—I vaguely remember her.
The Defense: What do you remember?
The Witness: Well, I remember from the punishment I was given at the time.
The Defense: What was happening to you?
The Witness: It was two of us and she was constantly whooping us and putting us down in the basement and that is where we spent all our time until they moved me from her home to another home in Georgetown and I remember that. We didn't stay there long because we went to Mrs. Hawkins' house.
The Defense: How old were you when Mrs. Hawkins started looking after you?
The Witness: I was about—about nine years old, I think.
The Defense: Would it be correct it might have been eight or nine?
The Witness: Yes.
The Court: He stated nine. Let him testify, sir.
The Defense: Now, did Mrs. Hawkins send you to school?
The Witness: Yes, sir, she did.
The Defense: Did you learn to read and write?
The Witness: No, sir, I didn't.
The Defense: Why not?
The Witness: Well, I used to be on my way to school but I—somewhere I didn't like the surroundings of school and I didn't like the children and things and I didn't go.

I stayed in the parking place and I didn't go to school.

THE DEFENSE: Why didn't you like the children at school?

THE WITNESS: It seems I wouldn't get along. I was more confused. I don't know.

THE DEFENSE: Did there come a time, . . . when you were sent to any special school?

THE WITNESS: I was sent to a boy's school, Blue Plains and I stayed there for a while and down there—

THE DEFENSE: Can you remember the name of the school?

THE WITNESS: It was Incorrigible School for Boys.

THE DEFENSE: And did you learn to read and write there?

THE WITNESS: No, sir, I didn't.

THE DEFENSE: What did you do when you returned from the school for incorrigible boys?

THE WITNESS: Well, I went back to Mrs. Hawkins' home and she put me back in school but I still didn't continue. I didn't go to school too much.

THE DEFENSE: Why didn't you go to school too much?

THE WITNESS: I played hookey a lot and I didn't—I just didn't like being in school. I didn't like the crowd in school. That's all.

THE DEFENSE: When you say you didn't like being in school, what was it that bothered you? . . .

THE WITNESS: Well, it seems as though I couldn't explain. I just started out to school and never got there. I would be by myself, you know. I just didn't make it to school. . . . .

THE DEFENSE: Well, what happened then? . . .

THE WITNESS: Well, I finished—I came out of school and I was sixteen and I—

THE DEFENSE: Were you able to read or write?

THE WITNESS: No, sir.

THE DEFENSE: What happened at that stage?

THE WITNESS: Well, I got a job as a messenger and put my age up for the job as messenger and that caused me to be drafted into the service.

THE DEFENSE: When you say you put your age up, . . .

what do you mean by that?

THE WITNESS: I said I was eighteen but I was only seventeen. I went in the service.

THE DEFENSE: What year?

THE WITNESS: It was in '42.

THE DEFENSE: How did you make out in the Military Service?

THE WITNESS: Well, I didn't make out too good.

THE DEFENSE: What happened to you?

THE WITNESS: I become to having headaches in the service and they put me in the hospital and I stayed there and they discharged me from the hospital.

THE DEFENSE: Do you remember what kind of a ward you were in when you went to that Army Hospital?

THE WITNESS: It was a mental ward.

THE DEFENSE: What did you do upon your discharge Mr. . . . [Rivers]?

THE WITNESS: Well, I came out of the service and I was walking down—about a week after I was out of the service, I was walking down the street and a fellow shot out of the door at another fellow and hit me behind the leg and I went to Casualty Hospital and I lost my leg after that.

THE DEFENSE: How did you happen to lose your leg?

THE WITNESS: Well, gangrene set in my leg and they had to take it off.

THE DEFENSE: And what did you do after being discharged from the hospital?

THE WITNESS: I stayed in the hospital a month and I went home.

THE DEFENSE: What was home to you at that time?

THE WITNESS: Mrs. Hawkins. Then I used to go out at night. I didn't like to go out in the day time and I used to go out at night more or less and I didn't want to associate with anybody after I lost my leg.

THE DEFENSE: Why didn't you like to go out in the day time?

THE WITNESS: People would be nosing you and every friend I had, they asked me what had happened and I just didn't like to be bothered too much with things like that and I used to go in the park and sit down and sit with another fellow that I knew.

THE DEFENSE: What did you feel during that period?

THE WITNESS: Oh, I felt like everything was at the end then for me. I had two strikes against me. I felt I had been mistreated. I don't know.

THE DEFENSE: What were you thinking about?

THE WITNESS: Well, at that time I didn't care what would happen, if I killed myself or what happened.

THE DEFENSE: Did there come a time when you met someone on a park bench?

THE WITNESS: I met a fellow that I had known before I went in the service and him and me used to always talk and be about together and so he was using drugs and that's when I began and I got interested and he showed me where it wouldn't hurt me and that's when I started using drugs.

THE DEFENSE: Why did you start using drugs, Mr. . . . [Rivers]?

THE COURT: He said it wouldn't hurt him.

THE DEFENSE: Was there any other reason why?

THE WITNESS: With him he was a friend and I accepted everything that was said and I wanted to do something to at least—I accepted him.

THE DEFENSE: What did you think the drugs would do to you when you took them?

THE WITNESS: It would make me—I don't know at the time I taken them exactly what it would do but after I taken them I felt all right.

THE DEFENSE: How did they make you feel?

THE WITNESS: They made me feel very good. They made me feel like I was living again. They made me feel pretty nice.

THE DEFENSE: And you didn't feel that way without the drugs?

THE WITNESS: No. Before I started using drugs, I used to have trouble with my leg, pain, and I felt as though I had my leg but my leg was off. I used to reach down and scratch my leg and my leg wasn't there and when I started using drugs, this left and all.

THE DEFENSE: And you have used drugs ever since?

THE WITNESS: Yes, ever since.

THE DEFENSE: How did you feel when you did not have any narcotics?

THE WITNESS: Well, if I didn't have any narcotics, I would feel sick. I would feel—I didn't feel the same as I did when I had narcotics. I would feel different. It wasn't —just feel out of place.

THE DEFENSE: In what way?

THE WITNESS: In all ways, all ways. Just feel out of place. You know, I didn't feel right. That's all.

THE DEFENSE: What did you do to prevent running out of drugs?

THE WITNESS: Well, I did—I stole. I committed various crimes to have money to get drugs.

After recounting a protracted criminal career based entirely upon the urge to secure drugs, the defendant went on to recall:

> ... I got a job and I was on that job and I had been away for three years and coming down the street I just taken—I started using drugs and I got disgusted with myself and so I come down the street and I taken a brick and throwed it into the car and told the police to come and arrest me.

THE DEFENSE: Was anybody present when this happened?

THE WITNESS: Yes. The police was present.

. . . .

THE DEFENSE: Did anything happen to any of the people that you knew or loved around 1960?

THE WITNESS: Well, my—the lady that died, she was the one that raised me.
THE DEFENSE: What was her name?
THE WITNESS: Mrs. Hawkins she died.
THE DEFENSE: She died?
THE WITNESS: Yes.
THE DEFENSE: How did you find out about it?
THE WITNESS: Well, I was in—I was arrested at the time and the way I found out about it, another fellow he told me, he says, I seen your address in the paper where you lived and he said, your mother is dead. Everybody calls her my mother. He says, your mother is dead. I didn't believe it and so I went to the chaplain of the institution and he told me she was dead and I made them take me into town.
THE DEFENSE: Did anybody else tell you about it, your foster father?
THE WITNESS: He told me about it. He wrote me a letter and I had the fellows read it to me and he told me he didn't want me to come there any more because he figured I was the cause of her dying because she liked me so much and that I was more the cause for her dying and so I didn't go back there.
THE DEFENSE: What happened to you when you received this news?
THE WITNESS: So I just—when I came out, I went and got me a room in a hotel and got drugs and I taken—tried to—got all I could and I tried to—just put in a cooker and you know, just tried to kill myself. I tried to just lay down and die, you know, but that only—
THE DEFENSE: How much did you take?
THE WITNESS: I take two teaspoon fulls of heroin and morphine.
THE DEFENSE: Was that a lot more than you were usually taking?
THE WITNESS: Yes, sir, it was much more than I usually take.

THE DEFENSE: How much more?

THE WITNESS: Oh, that is a quite a lot more than I usually take.

THE DEFENSE: In terms of pills or capsules, how much more? You said you worked up to fifteen.

THE WITNESS: Out of a spoon you probably could get twenty pills out of a spoon.

THE DEFENSE: And you took how much?

THE WITNESS: I would say I taken a spoon full.

THE DEFENSE: Just one?

THE WITNESS: I had both heroin and—

THE DEFENSE: Two spoons?

THE WITNESS: Two spoons of it.

THE DEFENSE: What happened after that?

THE WITNESS: Well, it didn't kill me and so I was just confused and I just kept on shooting myself, kept on using it.

THE DEFENSE: You kept on using drugs?

THE WITNESS: Yes, sir.

THE DEFENSE: Did you keep increasing your dosage?

THE WITNESS: Yes sir.

Cross-examination left Rivers' testimony unimpaired.

As he left the stand and the court recessed for the usual fifteen minutes, I overheard a narcotics officer saying to the prosecutor:

"This is one of the craziest sob-stories I have ever listened to."

I recall the prosecutor's reply in approximately these terms:

"Crazy? Maybe. Sob-story? Yes. But don't underestimate its effectiveness."

Dr. Wilbur Hamman took the stand after the recess.

It became plain as he testified that he was handicapped by a lack of personal familiarity with the defendant. He also seemed half-hearted at times in supporting the proposition of drug addiction as a disease.

He had conducted a general evaluation of James Rivers' case primarily in the course of the diagnostic staff conference held at St. Elizabeths Hospital. Like the other members of the St. Elizabeths staff he had no knowledge of such facts in the defendant's life as the attempted suicide and the smashing of a window in the presence of a police officer. Moreover, Dr. Hamman's heavy reliance upon the hospital records and his lack of knowledge of the defendant as a human being tended to depersonalize his testimony and render it less compelling than it might have been.

He concluded that James Rivers had been suffering from a mental disease, on December 15, 1961 and that the crimes charged against him in his indictment were products of that disease.

He began by describing James Rivers as a man suffering from deepseated feelings of inadequacy and depression.

A hypothetical question asking him to assume the facts in Rivers' testimony followed.

Direct examination then proceeded as follows:

THE DEFENSE: Can you propound an opinion to a reasonable medical certainty as to the mental state of the individual described in this hypothetical situation?

THE COURT: Meaning by that whether he is suffering from a mental disease?

THE DEFENSE: Yes, Your Honor.

THE WITNESS: Based on that hypothetical question, I would say that he is, yes, suffering from a mental disease for many, many years.

THE DEFENSE: Can you describe the nature of this disease to us?

THE WITNESS: Only in broad terms since I am dealing with a hypothetical question. I would say that the characteristics that you described are that of a personality pattern disorder and by this I mean, in the recognized classification by the American Psychiatric Association, simply means that the pattern of the individual personality is disordered. He is ineffectual. He is self-defeating and I would also judge from the question, that this individual was a very anxious, tense and depressed type of individual who always felt things were going to turn out poorly for him and so feeling, usually provoked them so they did without being aware of it.

THE DEFENSE: Would you say an individual like that needed treatment?

THE WITNESS: Yes.

THE DEFENSE: What kind of treatment?

THE WITNESS: Well, on the basis of that question, it is rather hard to be more specific in terms of specific—what treatment would be effective, Mr. Arens?

THE DEFENSE: Would you be prepared to state that psychiatric treatment would be in order?

THE WITNESS: It would be in order but I don't know how effective it would be. It certainly should be tried.

THE DEFENSE: Can you describe this hypothetical person in the terms of the seriousness of the disease?

THE WITNESS: Yes. In view of the fact that his life adjustment has been so meager and again using the criterion of the American Psychiatric Association which breaks any disease to mild, moderate and severe, and the degree of severity with impairment, I would say this person is suffering from a severe disease. The disease is very severe.

THE DEFENSE: Now, Dr. Hamman, would you have an opinion as to whether an individual like this, like the one described in the hypothetical situation, would be prone to engage in the sale of narcotics as well as other illegal activities to maintain this habit?

THE WITNESS: This is a pretty common course of action of a person who becomes addicted and in order to maintain enough money to sustain his habit, he will sell in order to gain money for drugs. This is not unusual.

THE DEFENSE: I have no further questions. Thank you very much, Dr. Hamman.

Cross-examination of Dr. Hamman took close to two hours.

In essence, the cross-examination attempted to pinpoint the witness' diagnosis of inadequate personality, to show that the defendant was properly oriented and that he did not appear to manifest flagrant psychotic psychopathology and that, in brief, the defendant's symptoms did not rise to the dignity of a mental illness.

When I had talked to him outside the courtroom, on the morning preceding his testimony, Dr. Hamman had expressed the view that the average public hospital was in no position to treat narcotic addicts because the strain upon its facilities in the handling of more conventional forms of psychopathology was already great. He added that this made no more sense than the refusal to recognize beriberi as a disease in China before the turn of the century because of its wide prevalence and the lack of adequate facilities.

I had not sought any such explanation upon direct examination. However, upon cross-examination, Dr. Hamman responded to the suggestion, that James Rivers was the victim of a general underprivilege which could not be meaningfully related to a mental disorder, in these words:

> Well, the Chinese before the American scientists went over there were given polished rice and they developed beriberi and this was because they didn't have a good start in life and the American scientists went over there and gave them a good start in life and so I would agree with what you say in essence but this is border line and in a sense this is the reason for emotional disease.

On further cross-examination the court interjected and declared with emphasis:

> It is a fact that the hospital has certified, and you have a copy of it, I know, Mr. Arens, that this man is competent to stand trial and there is no mental disease.

In response to this, I moved for a mistrial and the court denied my motion.

As the court recessed, I was told that a senior member of the bar who had occupied a seat reserved for members of the bar during a part of the trial was suspected by court officials of signaling a defense witness—presumably with a view to influencing his testimony in favor of the defense.

Returning to my office on that day, I received a telephone call from Professor George Shadoan, the Director of the Georgetown Legal Intern Service. Professor Shadoan informed me that he had been contacted by a representative of a local daily newspaper. The reporter had told the professor that he had information that I had deliberately sought the displacement of a validly appointed counsel with a view to securing a fee for myself in this case. Professor Shadoan told me that it took a substantial amount of his time to persuade the reporter that I had no possible motive for pushing my way into the case and securing the displacement of counsel—particularly since this was an indigent case in which no fee was conceivable. He added that he believed that he had finally succeeded in making his point with the newspaperman, but concluded that he did not think that he had dispelled all doubts. He recounted that the newspaper reporter kept referring to the "Arens stable of psychiatrists."

THE SECOND DAY OF TRIAL—THURSDAY, JULY 5, 1962

The trial resumed on Thursday, July 5, 1962, and representatives of both the *Washington Post* and the *Daily News* began putting in appearances in the courtroom consistently thereafter.

Dr. Clotworthy was the first witness to take the stand for the defense that morning.

Youthful in appearance, Dr. Clotworthy was articulate and coherent. His persuasiveness, however, emerged solely from the dead letter of the transcript and not from his live testimony. The truth was, and Dr. Clotworthy was not certain of it until long after the smoke of battle had cleared away, that he had really not put his heart into winning the case to begin with.

Dr. Clotworthy had severe doubts as to whether available hospital facilities could provide any meaningful answer to the problem posed by the narcotics addict and expressed himself subsequently at a taped conference with fellow professionals as stating that he had somehow inexplicably become "infected by Arens' enthusiasm."

His feelings about this case have been most clearly revealed in a discussion with a colleague, when he exclaimed about James Rivers:

> He is a dope peddler and how much lower can you get than that?[10]

Although naturally soft-spoken, Dr. Clotworthy's answers from the witness stand came in frequent instances in near whispers, barely audible a few feet beyond the witness stand.

At starting, I elicited Dr. Clotworthy's professional opinion that ". . . [James Rivers] had been suffering from a mental disease on December 15, 1961 and that the crimes charged against him in his indictment were products of that disease."

I then inquired:

> Now, Dr. Clotworthy, would you tell the court and the jury how this mental disease which was discovered in this patient arose and how it developed?

---

[10] It is interesting that the note of moral condemnation in describing the "dope peddler" should be more prominent in the thinking of a psychiatrist than in that of the Assistant Director of the Federal Bureau of Prisons. The latter, Mr. H.G. Moeller, reported that the system of penal sanctions "in far too many instances, disregards individual differences which exist both between offenders and the character of their offenses. It tends to reduce to the same common denominator the rackets boss, his lieutenant and muscle men, the predatory pusher, the small trafficker whose involvement represents the need to supply his habit, and the socially inadequate victim of the abuse of drugs." Transcript of Proceedings, White House Conference on Narcotics and Drug Abuse, at 191 (1962).

Dr. Clotworthy responded:

... [James] does not know who his real parents were. His early life was spent being moved around from one foster home to another, homes that the Welfare Department would pay to take him in and feed him and take care of him and he went from one to another never finding a place that he felt like he was really cared for until he was about ten years old and at a time in these very early years when he should have been developing strength to cope with the hard knocks of the world, instead he was being beaten in one place or another place and whenever company came to the house, why, he was put down in the basement until the company went home.

He was never allowed to eat at the same table with the others in the family but he would have to eat some place on a box out on the porch and so that experiences like this tore him down rather than enabling him to grow and develop strengths like we all have needed in those early years.

Then when he went off to school, he was unable to learn to read or write. He had plenty of opportunity to learn but he was totally unable to learn this particular subject.

... this is [probably] a result of a block, a peculiar kind of block wherein one is simply unable to learn these things that come really fairly easily for people generally, and I have never seen anyone who had such a severe block in this respect that has lasted up to the present time and he can only write his name and that is about it and so as a consequence of these—of the early abuses, it resulted in this which has had a profound effect on his life because it is exceedingly difficult to get along in this world if you can't read or write and he felt very much out of place in the school, very embarrassed and humiliated that this was the case.

He found himself not going right to school but going right on by and off to fish or to watch a building going up or something like this and he got into trouble because of this, of course.

In 1945 a major event took place in his life which had an additional deteriorating effect on him and that was that he lost his leg in an accident and he would always—he always felt that one place he could be proud of himself was in his ability in sports and he was on some good football teams in the District here and when he lost his leg he felt like people were looking at him and he felt very different and very alone, as he said, 'I didn't want to be around anybody' and about a month after he got out of the hospital and he was sitting in the park wondering how this happened to him, why, someone came along and began talking with him and—he didn't feel very much at home with people generally, he didn't feel like he could really let his hair down with people very much but this person seemed to have a good bit in common with him and he was really able to sort of bare his soul to this person and he felt like he really had found a friend at this time when he was so much in need of a friend.

Unfortunately this person shortly after became—shortly after he had become acquainted with him said, you are feeling badly now about your legs and you have taken drugs at the hospital to relieve the pain, let me give you some drugs to make you feel better.

So he took him up on that and he has been on drugs ever since. Off of drugs he said only a week since that time, that is, not longer than a week, except for the times when he has been locked up in some institution of one kind or another.

He was depressed about losing his leg because he was turned down for jobs as a result of losing his leg and then with his craving for the drugs and feeling unable to get a job, then he resorted to stealing and getting money illegally in order to satisfy this craving and this craving is something which few of us have much conception of in which one feels that nothing in life is of any consequence except to gain the relief that comes from getting the drugs.

He then attempted to explain how he had gone about evaluating the history which he had obtained from James Rivers and in so doing remarked that he had been impressed with a sort of earnestness about his patient as he talked with him. To this, the judge responded that he was unable to follow him.

Dr. Clotworthy's obvious discomfort was intensified by his perception of some of the audience reaction. As he put it in a subsequent interview with a fellow professional:

> And the Treasury Department agent sitting there in the gallery, appalled at what you're having to say, as if you really were an enemy of theirs, that they go to all the trouble of trying to round up these guys only to have you try to get them out again.

Cross-examination sought to show that the defendant had not exhibited flagrant psychotic symptoms during his psychiatric interview and proceeded to pinpoint the doctor's diagnosis of sociopathic personality.

So insistent was the prosecution in its pursuit of this theme that I felt bound on redirect examination to inquire whether the doctor had ever encountered cases of mental illness not involving the hearing of voices or the seeing of visions. He answered in the affirmative and added that the bulk of his psychiatric practice consisted of the treatment of mentally and emotionally ill patients, devoid of auditory and visual hallucinations.

To all of the prosecution's questions upon cross-examination, Dr. Clotworthy replied in the barely audible whispers which had characterized his direct examination. If one bears in mind that Dr. Clotworthy was confronted with the booming baritone of the prosecutor upon cross-examination, one concludes that many of his responses which were only half-hearted were ineffective.

In a taped discussion with a fellow psychiatrist several weeks after the trial, Dr. Clotworthy manifested substantial ambivalence concerning his role:

> In participating one sort of gets caught up between an enthusiasm for winning the case and there is something about that that made me feel uncomfortable inasmuch as I wasn't wholeheartedly in favor of winning the case in a way, inasmuch as if he were acquitted on the basis of insanity and sent to a mental hospital it seemed to me highly unlikely that there would in the hospital be adequate facilities for really treating the guy sufficiently, effectively to enable him really to get back into society; that there would even be some question, if you had the most ideal circumstances conceivable for therapy, that it would be possible for him to go back in society. He had a certain number of assets which made me feel, 'Gee, it would be wonderful if he could get what he needs.'
> . . . .
> He was a guy that one could feel a lot of sympathy for, and yet, when you got right down to the cold hard practicalities of what he would be offered in the way of treatment it seemed very unlikely that society had much to offer him in the way of treatment. So, if he were sent to the hospital, then I would expect that, after some kind of gesture was made toward treating him, he would then be sent out, because the hospital would be evaluating him on the basis of whether he was psychotic or wasn't psychotic, and not being psychotic, why then he might be discharged at least, if I am aware of the facts, it wouldn't be reasonable to keep him in the hospital for the rest of his life. And yet, he would be a menace to society if he were able to leave in one year or five years or ten years, and as much of a menace as a psychotic person who society would feel quite justified in keeping

in for the rest of his life if he didn't get any better. So, there was a kind of enthusiasm for winning the case and yet *I couldn't exactly put my heart into something of this sort . . .*[11]

The third expert witness to be called by the defense was Dr. George Warren Sprehn.

Dr. Sprehn had been readily available for conferences in advance of trial and had expressed his appreciation of "the pre-planning with the defense attorney" which, in his view, "helped considerably in making the nature of response and explanations clear and pertinent."[12]

The opinion he expressed under oath, was that James Rivers was a victim of mental illness and that the crimes charged against him in the indictment were produced by that illness.

Asked to elaborate upon the development of James Rivers' mental illness on direct examination, Dr. Sprehn provided the following account:

> I think it would be well to go back to the beginning of his school career when for reasons of inhibition rather than lack of intelligence, he simply could not learn to read or write.
> This led to frustration on the part of the teachers and his foster parents to the point where he was eventually placed in an ungraded school and they just struggled along with him until he was sixteen and until he could leave school legally with what was considered to be the equivalent of a fourth grade education, without the ability to read and write.
> I might say that during that time he was also evaluated by the Child Guidance Clinic working for the Welfare Department at which time the placement of him in the ungraded school was recommended.
> Following his release from school, his only source of employment, as he put it, [was] odd jobs where he could use his physical abilities.
> He had long since given up hope of being able to use his head, as he put it, for anything that would be useful in gainful employment.
> . . . .

---

[11] Taped interview with fellow professional.
[12] Letter to counsel.

This was fine for him, I suppose, until—he said he upped his age to join the Army. Another attempt was made to teach him to read and write which failed but he got through the military service long enough to become honorably discharged and very shortly, within a matter of days after his discharge he was involved in some kind of shooting incident in which he sustained an injury to his leg which led to gangrene and an amputation and at this point he was left with a despairing feeling, that not only could he not use his head for anything as far as making a living but neither could he use his body any more and with a period of just despair and withdrawal, isolation and doing nothing until somehow he got himself involved with the taking of drugs and curiously enough through this was eventually sent to a reformatory, a prison, wherein in spite of his difficulties he did manage to learn something.

He became rather proficient as a dental technician and he became rather proficient in the art of tailoring and tests have established that he is capable of using his hands. However, even these efforts have been through his neurotic method of applying them and then turned into failure, frustration and defeat with the repetition of convincing himself that he was a worthless person. The utilization of any advantage in him—either from himself or from others, has repeated itself many, many times up to the present time.

Further direct examination produced this dialogue:

THE DEFENSE: What is the significance then of the criminal record which this defendant has acquired . . . ?

THE WITNESS: The repetition of the behavior which is ostensibly for the purpose of making his life better or giving him gratification but which in fact leads to a reduction in his self-esteem and reduction in his security and eventually dependence in terms of being a prisoner.

THE DEFENSE: What forces him into this repetitive pattern of self-defeat?

THE WITNESS: There are two things. One is the need to maintain some picture of himself as a worthless, no good person which repeats even currently. The other is to somehow, and this is the curious and very sick part of his behavior, somehow to contrive to repeat the pattern of self-defeat and failure with the eventual goal of acceptance and love.

THE DEFENSE: Can you explain this in more detail, Dr. Sprehn?

THE WITNESS: In his experiences early, the more miserable his state the more his chances of being recognized and accepted and taken care of and this pattern persisted at least until the age of eight and I think the overprotective attitude of his foster parents probably reinforced this, since the more he was protected, the more convinced he must have been that he was incapable of handling himself by himself, but at any rate, it is this notion, derived out of the experience, that the more worthless he makes himself the better his chances of acceptance and security are. This is the sick pattern of behavior.

THE DEFENSE: How does he view the possibility of imprisonment, for example?

THE WITNESS: Imprisonment for him is security and something that again confirms this earlier opinion of himself as a worthless and no good person which in spite of assets and evidence to the contrary, does not change his mind about himself.

THE DEFENSE: Now, Dr. Sprehn, would you proceed to trace the development of his mental illness for his later years?

THE WITNESS: Following his military service and the loss of his leg, he was befriended, if you like, by somebody who found or had narcotics available and involved him in the process of taking narcotics.

Here I would like to discuss a minute the process of becoming addicted to a narcotic. Narcotics have the peculiar effect of giving a sense of well-being, or relief of pain and I think many of you have had narcotics from time to time for that purpose without the loss of some feeling of self-esteem or self-respect. Hence, the repeating damage of the narcotic drugs, so to speak, to maintain this sense of relief of pain and a feeling of well-being so that the demand for the drug becomes increasingly great with exploitation by those who sell it with the eventuality that any step must be taken to procure money in order to obtain the drug and the steps he took as is well documented have been—involving him in robbery, housebreaking, sale of stolen goods and all of that, solely for the purpose of obtaining money to buy the drug to continue this state of relief of pain and anxiety together with the feeling of well-being.

. . .

The curious thing also about this is that if we want to consider that the drug gets a hold of a person, this man and others I have seen, too, have been able to give up the drug, have kicked it, as they put it, and have sustained varying periods without the drug, only at the point of some frustration, grief or disappointment in life, to go back in desperation with full knowledge of the self-destructive effect of it, taking it again, so the repeating pattern of self-destructive behavior in the face of frustration and anxiety must continue.

Here we have the drug effect and the personality disorder, mental illness working together towards the complete destruction of a personality.

There was one incident, where, for example, where having been released from Lorton Reformatory, he knew that if he stayed out on his own he would probably get back on drugs and he spotted a policeman and he picked up a brick and threw it through a man's window . . . and called the police and had himself arrested and he was immediately sent back to Lorton for a sentence and again to protect him, to care for him, and to keep this self-destructive impulse from manifesting itself to a greater degree.

Dr. Sprehn went on to recount James Rivers' attempt at suicide following the death of his foster mother.

Cross-examination followed what was by now a familiar pattern. After pinpointing the doctor's diagnosis, i.e., neurotic depressive reaction, with a view to disparaging it at a subsequent time as inconsistent with the diagnoses of the two preceding doctors, the prosecutor proceeded to elicit admission after admission that the defendant knew the difference between right and wrong and exhibited no flagrant symptoms of psychosis.

The court's participation in the questioning of Dr. Sprehn was substantial.

Dr. Sprehn had stressed the importance of "rapport" in the adequate diagnostic evaluation of any patient.

The judge asked Dr. Sprehn as to whether it was not likely that he was obtaining "rapport" from the defendant because he was a defense doctor as distinct from "some other doctor." The judge then asked him to assume that the defendant was lying when he had spoken of breaking a window in the presence of the police. When the doctor declined to accept this suggestion, the judge persisted:

THE COURT: Let me put it to you another way: Actually, wouldn't that be a good way to malinger?
THE WITNESS: Not the way he presented it. It is too logical.
THE COURT: Well, assume it not to be the fact.
THE WITNESS: You mean that he is telling me this to give me the impression that he is faking?
THE COURT: Yes, in substance.
THE WITNESS: Now, the fact of his doing that—the fact of his behaving as he said he did—
THE COURT: You and I have no rapport.

> Weeks after the event, Dr. Sprehn recalled his role in the case in these terms:
>
>> Under the expected courtroom tension . . . I found it difficult to conceptualize my thoughts on occasion, and was left with a feeling that I had not said exactly what I wanted to say. I noted a definite teamwork effort to elucidate the important data, and mild anxiety over the difficulty in accomplishing this through the question-answer technique. Cross-examination, on the other hand, consisted merely of a not too subtle attempt to attack and destroy both the logic and integrity of the witness. The well-known maneuvers, some of which I was alerted to ahead of time by Mr. Arens, were all there, contributing, as intended by the prosecutor, to a growing sense of exasperation and rage on my

part. I was reminded of the Communist propaganda technique where the provocateur is instructed to ask the same question, over and over again, in slightly different form, for the purpose simply to nettle the interrogated person. This kind of performance, with the audience of the jury, appears to me as a malignant contamination of the process of determining justice.

He put the matter differently but more succinctly in these terms:

> A prosecutor screaming at me from three feet away does not seem a favorable setting for the calm deliberation necessary to ascertain truth and administer justice.[13]

Dr. Sprehn's testimony concluded the defendant's case in chief.

As I left the courtroom that day for my office, I was told that one of my assistants had been physically removed from the witness room by a United States Marshal when she had attempted to convey messages to defense witnesses as to when they could be expected to testify.[14]

---

[13] A written report dated Oct. 11, 1962.

[14] Her memorandum of the events of Thursday, July 5, 1962 is self explanatory:

"Before court began that morning Mr. Arens asked me to call Dr. Sprehn and ask him to be at court at 10:45 A.M. He also gave me messages to convey to four witnesses as they arrived. I was to tell Mr. Hawkins, the foster father of the defendant, that he would not be called on to testify but to ask him to stay in the witness room until both Dr. Clotworthy and Dr. Sprehn had had an opportunity to discuss the defendant with him. I was to introduce both Dr. Sprehn and Dr. Clotworthy to Mr. Hawkins and ask them to talk to him. I was to discuss with Mrs. . . . [Rivers] the possibility that she was the defendant's second wife and that the defendant had not divorced his first wife before marrying her, and also to remind her that she must volunteer much of the details of her association with the defendant since Mr. Arens would not be able to ask her specific leading questions in court. I also asked Mr. Arens how I could contact him at counsel table. At first he said I could ask the U.S. Marshal to give him a note, but then said that was not feasible since the marshal was guarding the defendant and that I would have to come to the bar and attract his attention and that he would then come to me.

I was able to get a message to Dr. Sprehn after several attempts, and to give Mr. Arens' messages to Mr. Hawkins, Dr. Sprehn and Dr. Clotworthy during the early part of the morning session. However, when Mrs. [Rivers] arrived and I greeted her and accompanied her to the Witness

(Footnote continued on next page.)

THE THIRD DAY OF TRIAL—MONDAY, JULY 9, 1962

The trial was not resumed until the following Monday, July 9, 1962. On this day the prosecution presented its case in rebuttal of the insanity defense by calling two psychiatric witnesses.

To a participant-observer, experienced with the multiplicity of disagreements emerging from the testimony of medical witnesses representing the same side in personal injury actions, the synchronization of testimonial data by the St. Elizabeths physicians commanded respect as a feat of legal skill.

The first witness called by the prosecution in rebuttal of the insanity defense was Dr. Dorothy Dobbs of St. Elizabeths Hospital.

Dr. Dobbs had received her M.D. some six years earlier and had been on the staff of St. Elizabeths Hospital for two years.

She reported that the defendant had been committed to St. Elizabeths Hospital for a period of approximately ninety days.

She recalled that it had been "reported that Mr. . . . [Rivers had] made a very cooperative adjustment in the hospital and [that] he [had] presented no management diffi-

---

Room, I was interrupted by the U.S. Marshal before I could convey any message to her.

I was standing just inside the Witness Room with Dr. Sprehn and Mrs. . . . [Rivers] when the marshal appeared at the door and beckoned to us. When no one moved, he came into the Witness Room, *took me by the arm and led me out of the Witness Room, still without speaking a word.* Outside the Witness Room, he told me that I was to stay right out here (indicating the hall outside the Witness Room) and that I was not an attorney and was not allowed to talk to witnesses. I asked him if he knew I was working for Richard Arens, the defense counsel, and he said that the judge had said I was not to talk to witnesses when I was also listening to the testimony in the courtroom. I, of course, accepted his instruction from the judge."

She tendered her resignation to the project within a few days, explaining that the hazards attendant upon work with the project were more than she was willing to face.

culties whatsoever." She added that she had also been told that he "spent a fair amount of his time sleeping which is not unusual."

She concluded in answer to a question by the prosecuting counsel as to what the mental examination of the defendant showed "with respect to his demeanor or conduct" that "[it] showed that there was no unusual behavior ... no unusual mannerism and the patient answered the questions relevantly, that is, his answers were suitable to the questions." Further direct examination took this turn:

THE PROSECUTION: Was the patient alert?
THE WITNESS: He was alert.
THE PROSECUTION: Was he oriented, Doctor?
THE WITNESS: Yes, he was.
THE PROSECUTION: Was there any intellectual impairment of the defendant?
THE WITNESS: Well, his intelligence is slightly below average but not what I would call intellectual impairment.
THE PROSECUTION: Was his speech relevant and coherent?
THE WITNESS: Yes.
THE PROSECUTION: Was there any evidence of any delusion or hallucination, Doctor?
THE WITNESS: There was no such evidence.

The witness showed some familiarity with the background of James Rivers but was unaware of much of the data available to the defense psychiatrists.

In the light of her study of the case, she concluded that the defendant "did not suffer from a mental disease or defect on December 15, 1961."

Prosecuting counsel concluded his direct examination of the witness with the question as to whether "defendant ... was ... able to distinguish right from wrong on December 15, 1961."

The witness replied:

"In my opinion he was."

Upon cross-examination Dr. Dobbs conceded that James Rivers was not as "fit as a fiddle."

I asked her what was wrong with him, and she responded by pointing to the "history of the [defendant's] repeated antisocial behavior."

She conceded that James Rivers was a victim of drug addiction and that she did not regard drug addiction as "a healthy activity."

Asked as to whether it was not a fact that there was something wrong with every drug addict, she replied:

"Almost every one."

The following colloquy ensued, interrupted on a few occasions by the judge:

THE DEFENSE: Now, who are the exceptions?
THE WITNESS: This is difficult to be precise about, Mr. Arens. I can only talk about individuals one at a time usually.
THE DEFENSE: Does the medical literature refer to a normal drug addict outside of the hospital situation involving say, the terminal cancer patient or a patient that is being treated for a very severe physical illness and who is legitimately administered drugs to ease his pain?
THE WITNESS: I don't know if the literature uses the phrase a normal drug addict but certainly there are people such as you describe who are receiving narcotics.
THE DEFENSE: For what purpose?
THE WITNESS: For pain primarily.
THE DEFENSE: You do not know of a single mentally normal drug addict, do you, Dr. Dobbs, who did not sustain his drug addiction in the hospital setting and maintain it there?
THE WITNESS: I am having difficulty with the terminology, Mr. Arens. This, like all illnesses, is a relative matter.
THE DEFENSE: Mentally healthy drug addicts, Dr. Dobbs. I would like to oblige.
THE WITNESS: Thank you. I have seen on occasions drug

addicts, as I have testified already, whom I do not regard as mentally ill although, obviously, they are not, as I stated, ideally mentally healthy people.

THE DEFENSE: Leaving the ideal aside for a moment, Dr. Dobbs, have you ever seen a mentally healthy drug addict who did not sustain his addiction in the course of legitimate administration of narcotic drugs for a physical illness?

THE WITNESS: I am sorry, Mr. Arens, I am having difficulty answering the question, obviously, because of this mentally healthy or mentally sick. They are not that extremely separated.

THE DEFENSE: There are gradations of gray between black and white, is that correct?

THE WITNESS: Yes.

THE DEFENSE: Would you tell us something about these gradations?

THE COURT: In what respect, sir?

THE DEFENSE: I am not sure that I understood the witness's response to my last question. I am seeking further information. She said they are not extremely separated.

THE WITNESS: That is correct.

THE DEFENSE: Thank you, Dr. Dobbs. I am now trying to establish what lies between the obvious blacks and the obvious whites, subject, of course, to the Court's permission.

THE COURT: Of course, if you can answer the question, Doctor.

THE WITNESS: I shall attempt a more or less hypothetical illustration. Well, I have seen such patients. Let us take, for example, a feeling of inadequacy. At one extreme we might have patients who literally believe themselves to be almost microscopic in size or to be the most worthless and blameworthy people on the face of the earth and—

THE DEFENSE: People who said good-bye to reality, is that correct?

THE WITNESS: Yes, I think so.

THE DEFENSE: All right.

THE WITNESS: On the other extreme, if I may continue, the ordinary every day, let us hope, normal population who now and then will have twinges of feeling that I am just not quite up to the job I have to do today.

THE DEFENSE: Now, you are not classing this man as the normal, everyday individual citizen who has occasional twinges which make him feel he is not quite up to the job that he has to do today, are you?

THE WITNESS: No, I don't suppose so, although—

THE DEFENSE: Now, Doctor—

THE COURT: Have you finished?

THE WITNESS: I was about to say that one might hypothesize certain feelings of inadequacy, for example, as in Mr. . . . [Rivers]. I do not recall that he made specifically such a statement in my hearing.

THE DEFENSE: Now, how long did you examine Mr. . . . [Rivers], Dr. Dobbs?

THE WITNESS: As I stated, on the occasion of the staff conference, I would estimate he was in the room approximately forty minutes.

THE DEFENSE: Do you regard this as a completely adequate mental examination?

THE WITNESS: I regard it as adequate, yes.

Dr. Dobbs admitted that the psychologists had labeled James Rivers as an "emotionally unstable personality" upon the basis of their tests at St. Elizabeths Hospital and that that particular diagnostic label was included in the American Psychiatric Association's *Diagnostic and Statistical Manual* as a mental disorder.

Cross-examination at this stage sought the sources of her background information on the patient:

THE DEFENSE: Madam, did you write a letter to the District Attorney or did the St. Elizabeths physician in charge of the study write a letter to the District Attorney requesting information about this case?

THE WITNESS: I believe so. We do it routinely.

THE DEFENSE: Do you also routinely write letters to the defense counsel inquiring as to what information he has?

THE WITNESS: Not usually.

To this, there was instant reaction from the bench:

THE COURT: There is a very good reason for that, sir. That is a privileged condition, sir, and you have no right to get it from attorneys.

I requested a bench conference and when that was granted, discovered that I had launched some not inconsequential developments with an objection to the court's comment in this way:

THE DEFENSE: I object to the Court's comment on this specific point.

THE COURT: Certainly, but it is a fact, isn't it?

THE DEFENSE: No, Your Honor, they could request a waiver of the privilege.

THE COURT: From an incompetent person, sir?

THE DEFENSE: On numerous occasions I have offered to make information available and the only reason I did not in this case was because I got into this case very late.

THE COURT: When did you get into this case, sir?

What followed was a judicial inquiry consuming eight and a half pages of the official transcript into the manner by which I had entered the case which was now on trial.[15]

The suggestion was clear-cut that I had succeeded in securing the displacement of another lawyer for improper

[15] It must be recalled that this inquiry following directly upon the heels of an objection to a judicial comment which was clearly erroneous came at the climax of the cross-examination and effectively destroyed any psychological advantage which I might have gained in the cross-examination of that witness up to that point.

purposes and in violation of the law.[16] I had done so moreover, in the view of the court, in a case which savored of the worst in litigation. As expressed by the court:

> ". . . I know of many assigned counsel who would not have taken the case on a retainer because they would not get into that type of case . . ."

When, upon recross-examination, Dr. Dobbs was asked as to whether James Rivers would be denied help by a "good psychiatric clinic" if he said he wanted help, the court refused to permit an answer, adding:

> Anybody that wants to pay for the service would get it, as you Ladies and Gentlemen well know.

The second psychiatric witness in rebuttal of the insanity defense, called by the prosecution, was Dr. David Owens.

Dr. Owens identified himself as a graduate of a medical college in 1948. He had had a one year internship, followed by approximately three years of private practice. He stated that he then served in the Army Medical Corps for two years. He came to St. Elizabeths Hospital in 1955 and was at the time of his testimony the Clinical Director of the John Howard Pavilion.

He testified that while he did not remember the exact number of psychiatric examinations he had performed, it was "up in the thousands."

Dr. Owens' background information on the patient was substantially the same as that furnished by Dr. Dobbs. Significantly, unlike Dr. Dobbs, who had clearly stated that St. Elizabeths Hospital did not routinely obtain information from defense lawyers, Dr. Owens claimed reliance on "information from lawyers, his attorney from the court, the District Attorney."

---

[16] It is noteworthy that the counsel for the prosecution was not interrupted once throughout the extensive proceedings held within the District Court.

Dr. Owens then described the patient in these terms:

"I am aware that he made an excellent adjustment while in the hospital. He had no difficulties. He got along well with the other patients."

Asked as to whether the patient had engaged in "any unusual or strange conduct . . . during his stay in the hospital," Dr. Owens replied in the negative.

In the light of all of the information available to Dr. Owens, including knowledge of the defendant's drug addiction, Dr. Owens stated that it was his professional opinion that James Rivers was without mental disorder on December 15, 1961.

He conceded that the patient showed "symptoms of . . . mental illness . . ." but as he viewed them, the symptoms did not warrant a diagnosis of mental illness. This is how he put the matter:

> There were certain—what we call sociopathic or antisocial acts which are committed against society, such as criminal acts On occasions repetitious acts of this nature are considered to be of a sociopathic type personality. . . . However, the symptoms that he displayed were not—it was mainly the history that we obtained and I didn't believe as a result of my examination, that the symptoms were of a sufficient severity to say that this is a mental disease because it was mainly obtained from the history of the patient, previous difficulties and not as a result of my examination.

Dr. Owens' direct examination by the prosecuting counsel was then terminated on what was now a familiar theme:

THE PROSECUTION: Doctor, in your opinion was the defendant . . . able to distinguish right from wrong on December 15, 1961?
THE WITNESS: Yes.
THE PROSECUTION: In your opinion, Doctor, could the defendant . . . embrace the right and resist the wrong?
THE WITNESS: In my opinion I would say that he could . . .

The following admissions, however, were secured from Dr. Owens upon the subject of the closeness of his contact with the patient on cross-examination:

THE DEFENSE: Now, Doctor, does it not happen in the course of psychiatric practice that an initial diagnostic impression is made on the basis of preliminary contacts and that impression is then subsequently revised when an intimate and intensive psychiatric relationship is established with the patient?

THE WITNESS: Yes, I think this happens, yes.

THE DEFENSE: You did not establish an intimate and intensive psychiatric relationship with this patient, did you, Dr. Owens?

THE WITNESS: No, I don't think anybody could in three months time.

THE DEFENSE: In three months time?

THE WITNESS: Yes.

THE DEFENSE: You never even bothered sitting down with him and saying, what is troubling you, . . . ?

THE WITNESS: Well, I didn't do it alone. As I indicated to you it is not required to be alone with the patient in order to establish some type of rapport with him but I did not examine him alone.

Questioned as to the adequacy of his study, Dr. Owens asserted that his psychiatric examination of the patient met the standards set forth by Dr. Karl Menninger in his book, *A Manual for Psychiatric Study*.

The line of inquiry proceeded as follows:

THE DEFENSE: [I]s this man . . . [Rivers] an emotionally healthy person?

THE WITNESS: In my opinion he is.

THE DEFENSE: An emotionally healthy person?

THE WITNESS: Well, I am saying he has no mental disease and therefore he is healthy emotionally.

I proceeded to question Dr. Owens as to the standards of emotional health, furnished by the American Psychiatric Association in its *Glossary,* as applied to this case:[17]

These were the questions and answers:

THE DEFENSE: Has . . . [Mr. Rivers] achieved reasonably satisfactory integration of his instinctual drives?
THE WITNESS: Yes I think he has. . . .
THE DEFENSE: Has his integration been acceptable to himself and to his social milieu as reflected in the satisfactory nature of his interpersonal relationships?
THE WITNESS: I think his interpersonal relationships have been satisfactory. . . .
Yes, I would say so.
THE DEFENSE: Now, sir, has he achieved . . . satisfaction in . . . living?
THE WITNESS: I don't think he has maintained the maximum satisfaction of living. I don't think any of us have and I think his is probably to a lesser degree than to most people.
THE DEFENSE: . . . And finally, if you please, has he attained . . . adequate achievement, flexibility and emotional maturity?
THE WITNESS: I think he has.

Dr. Owens admitted that he had no knowledge of such background data as Rivers' attempted suicide as well as his destruction of the window pane in the presence of a police officer. The fact that such data had been communicated to defense psychiatrists as distinct from the psychiatrists at

---

[17] The American Psychiatric Association Glossary defines emotional health as "a state of being which is relative rather than absolute in which a person has effected a reasonably satisfactory integration of his instinctual drives. His integration is acceptable to himself and to his social milieu as reflected in the satisfactory nature of his interpersonal relationships, his level of satisfaction in living, his actual achievement, his flexibility and the level of emotional maturity which he has attained."

St. Elizabeths Hospital struck him, he declared, as suggestive of malingering:

> The reason this individual relates this information to some people and some he does not, usually this is pretty indicative of further investigation on the part of the individual. If he tells you that he attempted to commit suicide and doesn't tell me, then I would certainly question the motives of why he had been holding information from me and giving it to you or vice versa.

Dr. Owens insisted that he had known a number of individuals chronically addicted to drugs who were without mental disorder:

I then asked him:

> Dr. Owens, can you provide us with a description of a normal, mentally normal chronic narcotics addict?

Dr. Owens replied, pointing in the direction of the defendant, who was then resting slumped over his chair, his eyes half-closed, but focused on the floor in what appeared to be abject depression:

> I think this is one.

This was about the best that I could do in eliciting a description of the normal chronic narcotics addict—discoverable apparently only upon the premises of St. Elizabeths Hospital. A further attempt at probing this concept of mental health was frustrated by action from the bench:

THE DEFENSE: I have asked you before, sir, can you describe the typical addict—
THE COURT: Don't repeat, sir.

Dr. Owens then interpreted the *Diagnostic and Statistical Manual* of the American Psychiatric Association as failing to list drug addiction as a mental illness.

Queried about the definition of sociopathic personality in

the *Diagnostic and Statistical Manual,* Dr. Owens declared that James Rivers' profile was not sociopathic because his "adjustment had been satisfactory other than in drug addiction."

THE DEFENSE: And do you call six convictions a satisfactory adjustment in terms of society?
THE WITNESS: Well, I will say this: You mean six convictions for drug addiction or other convictions also?
THE DEFENSE: Six convictions for criminal offenses and ... I believe, one or two including drug addiction.
THE WITNESS: Well, I don't think that criminal offenses in and of itself, whether it be six or sixty necessarily means just because an individual has so many criminal offenses that this is equal to mental illness. I think this is quite often indicative of some maladjustment in the individual but not always does it mean that because a man is convicted or is charged with a number of criminal offenses that therefore he is mentally ill.

This concluded the prosecution's rebuttal testimony. Dr. Randolph Frank was called as a rebuttal witness for the defense that same day.

Dr. Frank had taken on the limited job of the evaluation of the St. Elizabeths Hospital records. He had refused to examine the patient in person and claimed to have spent some two and one-half hours in a study of the hospital records.

His grasp of the details of the records, however, appeared clearly less than mine and I had not spent in excess of one-half hour in perusing them.

The doctor's appearance on the witness stand was, moreover, embarrassing.

Throughout some of his testimony, he could be observed rocking about in the witness chair with his eyes fixed upon the ceiling.

When he looked in the direction of the jury, it was at times with what appeared to be a smile, half-embarrassed, half-triumphant, accompanying such observations as that the defendant's loss of a limb had a definite symbolic significance to him as a psychiatrist.

He characterized the St. Elizabeths records he had studied as reflecting inadequate diagnostic procedures as well as "glaring inconsistencies."

He proceeded to express his "understanding and belief" that "only people that are accidentally addicted in the course of a chronic illness following an operation might be considered accidental addicts or medical addicts . . . [but that all other addicts are] chronically ill emotionally."

On three separate occasions, closely linked together, the trial judge asked Dr. Frank whether he was saying that "drug addiction alone without more . . . is listed as a disease." Each time the judge received an affirmative answer. The judge then asked the same question again, receiving the same response. Within minutes the judge asked substantially the same question for the fifth time and received the fifth affirmative response.

Dr. Frank concluded his testimony on direct examination but not his testimony on cross-examination at the end of that day's session.

Tuesday, July 10, 1962

No court was held in the *Rivers* case on Tuesday, July 10, 1962.

That day I was in the courthouse on another case. As I hurried to enter the courtroom a few minutes before a case was to be called, I was stopped by Dr. Owens. He and several of his colleagues were passing the time in conversation in a courthouse corridor while waiting for *their* cases to be called.

Dr. Owens asked me why the *Rivers* case was still on.

I replied that the *Rivers* case was still on because a defense psychiatrist had not yet finished testifying as to the inadequacy of the St. Elizabeths diagnostic work-up.

Dr. Owens demanded the name of the offending psychiatrist. I replied that he could obtain his information from his usual source, the office of the United States Attorney.

Dr. Owens appeared visibly upset. He said that I had made a "very nasty" statement.

An angry exchange followed. I inquired if Dr. Owens really believed in the mental health of the narcotics addict. He inquired as to where I had received my degree in psychiatry. I retorted that the best means of securing an authoritative resolution of this clash of viewpoints was by sending a transcript of his testimony to the American Psychiatric Association, and that this was what I proposed to do.

Conversation stopped at this point.

Late in the evening of July 10, 1962, I received a confidential telephone call informing me that Dr. Owens, after consultation with Dr. Mauris Platkin and Dr. Winfred Overholser, had filed a formal complaint with the United States Attorney's office that I was intimidating him and his staff.

THE FOURTH DAY OF TRIAL, WEDNESDAY, JULY 11, 1962

Prior to the commencement of the court session, Doctors Owens and Platkin could be seen stern-faced, pacing the courthouse corridor adjoining the courtroom. As soon as the marshal gave the first indications that the court was about to convene, both doctors seated themselves conspicuously in some of the spectators' seats.

The courtroom had filled rapidly with members of the bar including the principal Assistant United States Attorney, a Georgetown University law professor, the president of the Washington School of Psychiatry and the director of research on mental examinations of the Judicial Conference for the D.C. Circuit.

A bench conference was requested by the prosecuting counsel, who proceeded to inform the court that I had engaged in an act of intimidation against Dr. Owens. The claim was one of technical intimidation in the sense that Dr. Owens, although not handicapped in this case insofar as his testimony had been concluded, was subjected to the threat of the hostile scrutiny of the American Psychiatric Association in the future and might thus be inhibited in other litigation.

The judge dropped the matter after suggesting that in his view this involved an extremely serious transgression. His major concern appeared over the purported attempt to transmit any part of the transcript to the A.P.A. I assured him that in view of his feelings nothing would be sent to the A.P.A. He replied that this was a decision which must be dictated by my conscience rather than by any order by the court.

As the bench conference ended I became aware of the fact that the Fourth Estate, represented again by newspapermen from the *Washington Post* and the *Daily News,* had put in another appearance after having missed a day before this. The newspaper reporters left promptly upon the termination of the bench conference.

At the conclusion of the bench conference, Dr. Frank resumed the witness stand.

At the termination of his testimony, he was summoned—in full view of the jury—to the bench to answer questions concerning his fees and professional associations.

He had been subjected before this to a battery of forty-seven questions by the trial judge.

What followed was a roving inquisition into the corporate structure of the Washington School of Psychiatry, which had been instrumental in securing the witness, the fee arrangement approved for the witness, and the dependence of defense counsel's salary upon the trial of any specific number of cases.

Part of the judicial questioning at that stage was addressed to my status under the research project which contemplated the trial of a number of cases. The judge was not content with establishing the source of payment for both counsel and psychiatric expert witnesses. The question was repeatedly put to me as to whether my remuneration for N.I.H. research was "dependent" on the trial of a number of cases.[18]

No further witnesses were called.

Mr. Kenneth Schroeder, however, appeared in court to answer a protracted and hostile judicial inquiry, starting with this admonition:

> Now Mr. Schroeder, when you are appointed by the court and you for any reason feel you are not competent or for any other reason do not desire to serve, you should come back to the court and ask to be relieved. You have no authority to delegate to other people the case.

Mr. Schroeder replied:

> My position . . . was this . . . I was court appointed counsel . . . and I interviewed the defendant . . . the defendant confided in me at the time that he thought he was sick and needed help and I said I would do everything that I could to help him. He was indigent and we had no funds in the Georgetown Legal Intern Program to help him and I made the appropriate motion

---

[18] The following question arises on reflection upon the court's action in this matter.

The details sought after included the type of check by which an expert witness was paid, the manner in which the check was routed to him, his professional associations, and the membership of the board of directors of the Washington School of Psychiatry.

It is not perhaps irrelevant to note that at about this time and for some time thereafter, informal charges of solicitation of cases leveled against me in open court as well as outside the courtroom were founded upon the proposition that if I was "employed" by N.I.H. and/or the Washington School of Psychiatry to try a given number of cases, this employment obviously was contingent upon such trial and my request to Legal Aid or anybody else to secure indigent cases constituted a form of soliciting which not only was unethical but rendered me liable for champerty and barratry.

to send the defendant to St. Elizabeths which was granted and after observing the defendant for a period of ninety days, the report came back that he was mentally competent. I went back and [so] informed the defendant . . . He expressed . . . dissatisfaction to me with the procedure at St. Elizabeths. At that time I felt not only obligated under the canons to believe him but I also had my own personal views on the procedure at St. Elizabeths.

He asked me if there was anything further that could be done. . . .

Once again I felt that I was morally obligated under the canons to seek help elsewhere . . . I knew of Mr. Arens' program and I maintain . . . that I had an obligation to seek that help.

Mr. Arens had the staff and the money under his program to give . . . assistance. I explained the procedure to Mr. . . . [Rivers] and I told him that Mr. Arens was a competent attorney which is evidenced by his presentation of this case in court and told Mr. . . . [Rivers] that he could probably get better help from him and his staff . . . and Mr. . . . [Rivers] agreed to let Mr. Arens handle the case.

The day concluded with a conference in chambers on the proposed instructions, submitted respectively by the defense and prosecution.

In view of the nonpsychotic nature of James Rivers' mental disorder and in view of the prosecutor's stress on the basic integrity of his cognitive functioning, I attempted to secure instructions to the jury which would make it crystal clear that the popular concept of the conventionally insane person was inapplicable and that an acquittal by reason of insanity was in order even if the defendant did not match the popular conception of the lunatic and even if he knew the difference between right and wrong.

Almost simultaneously with the *Rivers* trial, the Supreme Court ruled in *Robinson v. California* that a sovereignty had no power to punish an individual for the mere state of drug addiction. In so doing it noted that "counsel for the State recognized that narcotic addiction is an illness."[19]

---

[19] Robinson v. California, 370 U.S. 660 (1962).

It added:

> Indeed, it is apparently an illness which may be contracted innocently or voluntarily. We hold that a State law which imprisons a person thus afflicted as a criminal, even though he has never touched any narcotic drug within the State or been guilty of any irregular behavior, inflicts a cruel and unusual punishment in violation of the Fourteenth Amendment.[20]

I thought it mandatory under these circumstances to seek instructions as to the right of the jury to recognize narcotics addiction as an illness in the light of the Supreme Court opinion in *Robinson*. These requested instructions were denied.

Further discussion in chambers concerning other instructions proposed by the defense met a like fate:

THE DEFENSE: In this case, the contention was advanced by the defendant that he was not suffering from insanity in the conventional sense of the term, he was not hearing voices and he was not seeing things but nonetheless, we earnestly submitted to the court and the jury that he was mentally ill and entitled to acquittal on that score . . . and we believe . . . it would . . . prevent possible confusion among the jurors if the court . . . [would] state that to be entitled to acquittal by reason of insanity, the conventional concept of an insane person need not be considered binding.

THE COURT: They have not had a conventional concept to find for this jury and I think that you would be curtailing this man's rights by using it and polluting the stream by what is conventional and what is not. I intend to deal with it in a more basic manner and as I understand to be the law as given by the Court of Appeals, namely, if this man be suffering from a mental disease without regard to its label, . . . and if the act is a result thereof,

---

[20] *Id.*, p. 667.

then he is entitled to a verdict of not guilty by reason of insanity.

THE DEFENSE: I understand the court's position but I respectfully note an objection.

THE FIFTH DAY OF TRIAL—THURSDAY, JULY 12, 1962

The day opened with the *pro forma* renewal of the motion for mistrial on behalf of the defendant and the making of a motion for a judgment of acquittal by reason of insanity in the alternative.

Both motions were denied by the court.

In accordance with federal practice, the prosecutor had two turns at addressing the jury in his closing argument at the conclusion of the evidence, while the single closing argument for the defense was squeezed in between the two closing arguments for the prosecution.

The prosecutor's first address focused on the metaphysics of right and wrong, the doctrine of the infallibility of St. Elizabeths Hospital and the necessity of the punishment of the malefactor.

The malefactor, it was claimed, had established the categorical imperative for his punishment by demonstrating his ability to drive, work as a dental technician and as a tailor, as well as by functioning as an apparently "normal" human being.

The implication was plain that doctors who, notwithstanding such evidence of normalcy, chose to regard James Rivers as mentally ill, incurred the suspicion of all good men as to their motives and diagnostic standards.

Carried away by the heat of argument, the prosecutor evidently believed his own assertion that the doctors for the defense had based their diagnoses of James Rivers' mental illness on no more than his impoverished environment in early childhood and on the assumption that "all orphans are mentally ill." It was inevitable in this context that existing disparities in the diagnostic labels utilized by the psychiatrists who had testified for the defense were to be highlighted to show that such contradiction among psychiatrists on the same team rendered them unworthy of belief.

The following are representative samples in the development of the prosecutor's first argument:

> We have Dr. Hamman who was at St. Elizabeths Hospital and who participated in the conference and he diagnosed this man as an inadequate personality. He said his conclusions were based on the psychiatric interview, what the patient tells you, how the patient feels and other data.
>
> It was his opinion, Ladies and Gentlemen, that this defendant had the deep seated feelings of inadequacy and depression and you will note the way these doctors throw around terms and one doctor did say that it is very easy to be glib with labels because it makes an impression on people.
>
> Well, don't you be impressed by labels. You look for the facts and the reasons to support those facts because this man in Dr. Hamman's opinion had a feeling of inadequacy and depression and therefore he was an inadequate personality.
>
> Well, is there a person alive today, Ladies and Gentlemen of the Jury, that has a totally adequate personality? Everybody has feelings of inadequacy and is depressed. Does that make them mentally ill? If that is true, we have a lot of mentally ill people in this country.
>
> . . . .
>
> Now, Dr. Clotworthy is a man that says I think he is a sociopathic personality with drug addiction and depressive features and he talked to the defendant about an hour and a quarter. He said his diagnosis was based on poor childhood. He said his experiences in early years tore him down. How does Dr. Clotworthy know? Was he there? You get these concepts right out of the blue.
>
> . . . .
>
> Now, Dr. Sprehn comes in, Ladies and Gentlemen, and he diagnosed this man as a neurotic depressive reaction with sociopathic features. We have three doctors and we have three different directions. We are still in the field of personality disorders but we have three different diagnoses.
>
> The doctor tells you that his opinion doesn't depend on outside sources. He only looked at these sources afterwards.
>
> It was his view that this defendant was suffering from a mental illness on December 15, 1961. This is the same doctor who told you Ladies and Gentlemen that *all orphans are mentally ill.*
>
> Now, what kind of doctor is that? This doctor talks in terms

of self-defeatism. He says he has a predominant feeling of despair.
    These people look at the classic individual who should have a personality disorder and they decide he has some symptomatology which might be indicative of a mental illness and they say, Oh, he fits. That is where we will stick this man but what the doctors don't know, they all come up with different diagnoses.

When my turn came, I attempted to tell the jury that I would personally prefer being a schizophrenic with auditory hallucinations than a nonpsychotic drug addict, but I never got to say more than—"I would say that I would rather be a schizophrenic hearing voices than suffer—is that improper, Your Honor?" before the court interrupted:

You are not trying Mr. Arens at all.

The thrust of my argument was that James Rivers' ability to know the difference between right and wrong was irrelevant to an appraisal of his mental illness. I added that appropriate psychiatric evaluation of a patient like James Rivers depended upon rapport between the patient and the examining physician and that that rapport was more likely to be obtained by the doctors who had testified for him than by the busy staff of an overcrowded public hospital.
    I concluded:

There has been a great deal of talk addressed to you about his seeing no visions, his hearing no voices and again I say to you, . . . we have never claimed that he heard voices or saw visions. We say to you that he was mentally ill and I add that if mental illness depends upon the hearing of voices and the seeing of visions, we are back one hundred years in psychiatric thinking and I think you are too intelligent to put us that far back.

The prosecutor's rebuttal began with the specific denial of the proposition which I had urged as critical to the defendant's case.

Mr. Arens began by telling you, Ladies and Gentlemen, he was not concerned with the differences between right and wrong and whether this defendant, . . . was able to embrace the right and

> resist the wrong. I say to you, Ladies and Gentlemen, you are concerned with that. You are concerned with that because information of this nature is helpful to you as His Honor will indicate in determining whether this . . . [defendant] was suffering from any mental disease or mental defect on December 15, 1961.
> Wherein is a mental disease a mental defect if . . . [Rivers] did in fact know the difference between right and wrong and could exercise his volition in the direction of the right?

Addressing himself to the matter of rapport which I had raised, the prosecutor declared:

> The magic word rapport was used extensively by Mr. Arens. This is supposed to be some magic scheme whereby a doctor is able to better diagnose any possible illness a patient may have. Who is in a better position, Ladies and Gentlemen, to make the adequate diagnosis of . . . [James Rivers] the man who merely talked to him for a short period of time or the doctors who had the defendant under observation by themselves as well as others for ninety day commitment at the hospital?

Giving every appearance of genuine indignation, he referred to the testimony of all of the defense experts as "a shame [on] . . . the psychiatric profession" and to Dr. Clotworthy as the "unworthy Dr. Clotworthy."

Set forth *in extenso*, the prosecutor's argument on this score read as follows:

> Now Mr. Arens says that Dr. Clotworthy testified compassionately but impartially. This is a doctor, Ladies and Gentlemen, who said he couldn't think of a single thing the defendant said that was false. Not a thing and this unworthy Dr. Clotworthy said he makes mistakes on his diagnoses and he doesn't know much about drug addicts. How much credence can you put in the testimony of this doctor?
> Mr. Arens says the doctors didn't attempt to pull the wool over your eyes. I say to you that these doctors are label pinners. It is a shame to the psychiatric profession what you Ladies and Gentlemen have witnessed here this past week. You see doctors come down here, make a personal examination of an individual and say because he is a drug addict, because he had a poor childhood, because he never learned to read or write and suddenly he has a block and now he is an inadequate personality and others say he is a psychopathic personality, he is a depressive reaction type of individual with drug addiction and one even

said he is a mental defective and that doctor didn't even examine him. It is a shame on the profession.

My objection to this line of argument was brushed off by the court with the suggestion that this constituted proper argument.[21] Displaying reliance upon conventional conceptions of lunacy in rejecting the case made out for the defendant by his doctors, the prosecutor thereafter concluded:

> I say to you, Ladies and Gentlemen, putting . . . [James Rivers] in a mental institution will not be a proper place for him. Mental institutions, Ladies and Gentlemen, serve people who have mental illnesses as you and I know them.
>
> What . . . [he] really suffers from is a physical disability and you as a jury should tell the community that people who delve in drugs will be punished and not hospitalized.

The time had come for the court's charge to the jury.

The charge repeatedly invited the jury to disregard expert testimony not supported by sound reasoning. In view of the fact that only defense psychiatrists had been subjected to repeated cross-examination by the court suggestive of judicial incredulity, it was obvious that the court was inviting the rejection of the testimony of defense psychiatrists.

Thus in charging the jury, the court stated on five separate occasions that the jurors were not bound by expert testimony.

It did so in this manner:

> Now, an expert in a particular field is permitted to give his opinion in evidence but you are instructed that you are not bound by the testimony of such expert. . . .

---

[21] It is not unfair to observe that in permitting an attack upon the expert witnesses in the manner indicated, the court not only prejudiced the defendant's case but violated the existing legal rule governing jury arguments.

That rule can be summed up in these words:

"It is within the scope of proper argument of counsel to impugn the motives and assail the credibilty of opposing witnesses, *where the remarks are based upon evidence or reasonable inference therefrom.*" (emphasis supplied) Stevens v. Kasten, 342 Ill. App. 421, 423, 96 N.E. 2d. 817, 819 (1931).

In connection with expert testimony offered in this case, you should consider each expert's opinion received in evidence in the case and give to it such weight as you think it deserves and you may reject it entirely if you conclude that the reasons given in support of the opinion are unsound.

. . . The testimony of medical experts, psychiatric experts and their opinions should be weighed and considered by you in connection with all the other evidence in the case. You are not bound to accept the opinion of any expert as conclusive.

Where experts differ, it is for the jury to determine which expert testimony, if any, you should accept. The final decision is yours.

. . . .

You should consider the testimony of the different experts and weigh the reasons, if given, for their opinions. You are not, however, bound by such opinion. You may give to them such weight as you deem them entitled to and you may reject any expert testimony, if in your judgment, the reasons for it are unsound.

The court's charge as to the defense of insanity clearly and compellingly invoked the ghosts of lunacy of bygone days.

The opening note of the instructions on the insanity defense went as follows:

Now, this brings me to a matter of importance to all concerned, the question of mental capacity of this defendant, for in this case the defense has contended that the defendant was not sane at the time of the crime and that the act was the result of his insanity.

The government, on the other hand, contends that he was of sound mind at the time of the act.

Whether authorized under a literal reading of Court of Appeals opinions or not, the instructions given by the judge in this case seemed patently at odds with a liberal interpretation of the insanity defense at the time of the trial, as he further stated that:

The law does not hold a person criminally responsible if he is mentally deranged and his derangement causes him to commit a crime but it is not every kind of mental derangement or mental deficiency which is sufficient to relieve a person of responsibility for his acts. On the contrary, a person may suffer a mental abnormality and still be answerable for his unlawful acts.[22]

The judge provided but one explanation of what constituted a causal connection between crime and mental illness and this was:

> ... if a person at the time of the commission of a crime is so deranged mentally that he cannot distinguish between right and wrong or if able to tell right from wrong is unable by virtue of his mental derangement to control his actions, then his act is the product of his mental derangement.

---

[22] The impact of such instructions is more fully realized only if we recall the Judge's overt expression of skepticism or disbelief vis-à-vis the defense experts. This skepticism or disbelief was further revealed in the contrast in judicial questioning of defense and prosecution witnesses which lends itself to numerical tabulation.

There were five witnesses appearing for the government, three lay witnesses and two psychiatrists. For the defense, there was the defendant, four psychiatrists and the defendant's wife. Since the latter's testimony can be largely regarded as solely corroborative of the fact of the defendant's drug addiction, the Court's treatment of this witness would not appear critical and can be disregarded.

The trial judge asked a total of only one question of the three lay witnesses that appeared for the government. With respect to Dr. Dobbs, the government's first psychiatrist to take the stand, the Court asked her only one question and that was to bolster her testimony. The next psychiatrist to testify for the government was Dr. David Owens. The trial court asked him 10 questions, 9 of which clearly bolstered his testimony or assisted him generally. The 10th question restated the question asked by defense counsel in a way designed to bolster and support the witness. Thus the trial court asked the five lay and expert witnesses for the government a total of 12 questions.

The court's treatment of the defense witnesses was another story. The court asked the defendant 3 questions. The defendant's first psychiatrist, Dr. Hamman, was asked no less than 26 questions by the trial court. The next psychiatrist, Dr. Clotworthy, was asked a total of 15 questions. Next was Dr. Sprehn, who was asked 20 questions. And finally, Dr. Frank was asked no less than 47 questions by the trial judge.

Addressing oneself to the numerical aspect of judicial interrogation of defense witnesses one can say, in sum, that the trial court asked the 5 Government witnesses a total of 12 questions and asked the 5 defense witnesses (not counting the defendant's wife), a total of 111 questions, approximately 9 times as many.

In immediate juxtaposition to this statement of the *M'Naghten* rule, the Judge provided the further elaboration that "there . . . [was] a presumption of sanity . . . [and that every] person . . . [was] presumed to be sane until the contrary appears."

I noted the obvious objections to the charge.

A characteristic exchange between me and the court at a bench conference at this time went as follows:

THE DEFENSE: Your Honor stated that one of the examples of nonresponsibility under the law might be a situation where the individual did not know right from wrong. I think it is a perfectly accurate statement of law. I am concerned, however, . . . that the jury might assume that this is the only possible example. I was wondering if the Court could say there might be other examples as well.

THE COURT: I think it might be more confusing than helpful. I think I will leave it as it is.

The prosecution subsequently supported this position of the trial court before the Court of Appeals by asserting as a general principle that

> The judge was not required to supplement his insanity charge with specific negative instructions (1) that . . . [defendant] need not resemble a wild beast or be bereft of reason to be acquitted, and (2) that the right-wrong standard was not the *sine qua non* of acquittal.[23]

---

[23] *Cf.* The language of the Court of Appeals in Durham v. United States, 214 F.2d 262, 875, (D.C. Cir. 1954):

"We do not, and indeed could not, formulate an instruction which would be either appropriate or binding in all cases. But under the rule now announced, any instruction should in some way convey to the jury the sense and substance of the following: If you the jury believe beyond a reasonable doubt that the accused was not suffering from a diseased or defective mental condition at the time he committed the criminal act charged, you may find him guilty. If you believe he was suffering from a diseased or defective mental condition when he committed the act, but believe beyond a reasonable doubt that the act was not the product of such

(Footnote continued on next page.)

The jury retired at 12:23 P.M., and returned a guilty verdict slightly before 4:00 that afternoon.

POST TRIAL EVENTS

I met James Rivers again on sentencing day.

I spoke to him briefly in the cell block before sentencing. I informed him at that time, as I had before, that the minimum sentence he would face as a multiple narcotics offender was ten years. I added that in view of the atmosphere of the trial, we had to be prepared for a sentence which might be twice as long. Rivers swayed as though he had been struck a physical blow. He recovered rapidly, however, and proceeded to thank me for my services.

Brought before the bench, he received the minimum sentence of ten years imprisonment—coupled with a recommendation by the court that he be placed in a hospital unit of the federal prison system—but significantly without any possibility of parole under the terms of existing legislation.[24]

---

mental abnormality, you may find him guilty. Unless you believe beyond a reasonable doubt either that he was not suffering from a diseased or defective mental condition, or that the act was not the product of such abnormality, you must find the accused not guilty by reason of insanity. Thus your task would not be completed upon finding, if you did find, that the accused suffered from a mental disease or defect. He would still be responsible for his unlawful act if there was no causal connection between such mental abnormality and the act. These questions must be determined by you from the facts which you find to be fairly deducible from the testimony and the evidence in this case."

[24] If it is borne in mind that the penalty clauses of the Narcotic Laws represent revenue legislation and that James Rivers had evaded a *de minimis* amount of revenue due to the federal government his sentence clearly appears disproportionate to his offense. He, like other narcotics offenders of his kind, was sentenced to 10 years for a revenue law violation involving a loss to the government of only a few cents tax or duty. The severity of the sentence was further intensified by rendering him ineligible for probation or parole for the term of his sentence. It was compounded by the fact that it was imposed for a violation growing out of his diseased state. *Cf.* Robinson v. California, 370 U.S. 660 (1962).

An appeal was noted and a motion for leave to proceed without prepayment of costs granted by the District Court.

A faculty group at the Washington School of Psychiatry was at this time asked if it would be prepared to sponsor an *amicus* brief in support of the proposition that the psychiatric profession did not know of any chronic narcotics addicts—outside of restricted medical situations involving the legitimate administration of narcotics for physical pain—who were free of mental disorder. Members of the Washington School faculty, as well as every member of the "Arens stable of psychiatrists" met in conference on the Project on Law and Psychiatry at the Washington School. The senior members declined to sponsor such a brief. As I listened to the tape recording of the conference, I was struck by the fact that the psychiatrists who opposed filing an *amicus* brief, discussed the possibility of bringing a law suit against a prosecuting counsel who, they claimed, had implied that some of them had acted like "horse thieves" in another case.

A senior psychiatrist present at the conference, who had previously expressed his derision of the view that there was such a thing as a mentally healthy chronic narcotics addict, subsequently telephoned me to say that the conference had decided not to sponsor an *amicus* brief and that he was in no position to assert that the view of the chronic narcotics addict as mentally ill was "the generally accepted view in recognized schools of medicine as well as within every accredited institute of training and research in psychiatry in this country."

Independently of the Washington School of Psychiatry, Doctors Leo H. Bartemeier, Francis J. Braceland, Lawrence Kolb, William C. Menninger, Leon Salzman, and Winfred Overholser, among others, did not feel similarly incapacitated and declared in an *amicus* brief, filed in the Court of Appeals, that their view of the narcotics addict as mentally ill was indeed the "generally accepted view in recognized schools of medicine as well as within every accredited institute of training and research in psychiatry in this country."

A major surprise to both the defense and the prosecution was the fact that Dr. Winfred Overholser, who had retired as Superintendent of St. Elizabeths Hospital since the Rivers trial, now joined these *amici* in favor of the proposition which his hospital staff had resisted so vigorously when the case was in the trial court.

On the hearing of the case on appeal, a panel of the United States Court of Appeals spurned the major argument of the appellant. I had claimed before the Court of Appeals—consistently with the views expressed by the *amici*—that the contention advanced by Dr. David Owens that a chronic drug addict with James Rivers' history was mentally or "emotionally healthy" was as credible as the contention that the earth was flat. The court held that a jury issue had been presented, i.e., that the testimony of the St. Elizabeths' staff could indeed be believed by reasonable men. However, it found error in the fact that the trial judge had informed the jury that the St. Elizabeths staff had certified the defendant as competent to stand trial and remanded the case for a new trial accordingly.

CONCLUSION

Upon presentation of the mandate of the Court of Appeals, the United States Attorney's Office agreed to drop the two counts of the indictment under the federal narcotics statute and accept a guilty plea to a lesser included misdemeanor.

James Rivers was released on the basis of the time he had already served pending appeal. There is no reason to believe that a significant effort at medical or psychological rehabilitation had been made during that interval. Not too long after his release, James Rivers was again confronting a court on matters clearly linked to his previously demonstrated difficulties in living.[25]

---

[25] Since the time of the Rivers trial, Congress has given half-hearted recognition to the medical aspects of drug addiction by providing for the
(Footnote continued on next page.)

It is questionable whether the interests of the defendant or of society were served by what took place.

What is clear is that a lawyer defending a case of this kind may discover that he will be called upon to address himself, not only to the task of defending his client, but also to that of defending himself, and that his dependence on available psychiatric support will be precarious.

---

eligibility of some drug addicts, charged under the Federal criminal laws, for some measure of medico-psychological rehabilitation in *lieu* of criminal penalties. *See* Narcotics Addict Rehabilitation Act., 18 U.S.C. 4255 (1966).

The brutal cut-backs in the budgeting of rehabilitative institutions promised by that Act make it a snare, a trap and a delusion.

EPILOGUE

BACK TO METHUSELAH

THE BRAWNER DOCTRINE

Long after the conclusion of the Project, the Court of Appeals issued a formal death certificate for the *Durham* rule.

On June 23, 1972, it declared in *United States* v. *Brawner*[1] that the *Durham* rule was superseded by a new rule:

> "A person is not responsible for criminal conduct if at the time of such conduct as a result of mental disease or defect he lacks substantial capacity either to appreciate the criminality [wrongfulness] of his conduct or to conform his conduct to the requirements of the law."

The appellant, an epileptic, had been injured in the course of an altercation after a morning and afternoon of wine drinking. As seen by the Court, his "jaw was injured when he was struck or pushed to the ground" and he was subsequently described by lay witnesses as blurred in speech and looking "like he was out of his mind." The homicide with which he was subsequently charged was committed in that state.

On trial for murder, the accused asserted the insanity defense.

There was general agreement among the available experts, all drawn from St. Elizabeths Hospital, that the defendant had been suffering from a major mental disorder. He was

---

[1] ——F.2d—— (D.C. Cir. 1972).

uniformly viewed as an epileptic, suffering from "a mental as well as a neurological disease." A government physician—not unknown to the readers of these pages—testified, however, that the defendant's act of murder was not the product of an epileptic seizure nor that of the psychiatric disorder attributed to the defendant by the government doctors. "In the words of Dr. Platkin..., 'He was just mad' "—presumably in the non-psychiatric sense of the word.[2]

Dr. Platkin, it will be recalled, had once testified with comparable effectiveness under similar circumstances. Confronted with evidence that another defendant had attempted to throw his baby into a burning furnace and was prevented only by physical force from accomplishing this objective, he had declared that this was more suggestive of an "extremely vicious temper" than mental illness and that in fact it was not "evidence of mental illness" at all and did not "amount to mental illness" in any sense.[3] He had then gone on to discuss the phenomenon as a *normal* displacement of hostility.

[2] As summarized by the Court:
"All of the expert witnesses agreed that Brawner was suffering from an abnormality of a psychiatric or neurological nature. The medical labels were variously given as 'epileptic personality disorder,' 'psychologic brain syndrome associated with a convulsive disorder,' personality disorder associated with epilepsy,' or more simply, 'an explosive personality.' There was no disagreement that the epileptic condition would be exacerbated by alcohol, leading to more frequent episodes and episodes of greater intensity, and would also be exacerbated by a physical blow to the head. The experts agreed that epilepsy *per se* is not a mental disease or defect, but a neurological disease which is often associated with a mental disease or defect. They further agreed that Brawner had a mental, as well as a neurological, disease.
Where the experts disagreed was on the part which that mental disease or defect played in the murder of Billy Ford. The position of the witnesses called by the Government is that Brawner's behavior on the night of September 8 was not consistent with an epileptic seizure, and was not suggestive of an explosive reaction in the context of a psychiatric disorder. In the words of Dr. Platkin of St. Elizabeths Hospital, 'he was just mad.' "
United States v. Brawner, ——F.2d—— (1972).
[3] See Transcript of Proceedings, United States v. Willie Lee Stewart, *Crim.* No. 633-53, pp. 2049-2051-A (D.D.C. 1962).

Still in the *Brawner* case, a government psychologist had had the temerity to challenge the institutional judgment propounded by Dr. Platkin, by seeing meaningful evidence of exculpatory mental illness in the accused. This psychologist was subjected to a prosecutorial cross-examination followed by a prosecutor's summation, calculated at the least to demean the psychologist as devoid of professional qualifications.

Convicted on this evidence, the defendant appealed. In remanding the case to the trial court to consider whether a new trial was in order under a new rule of criminal responsibility—the Court of Appeals declined to find any problem of testimonial credibility and thus upheld the testimony of Dr. Platkin as capable of commanding belief among reasonable men.

As for the prosecutor's denigration of the psychologist, the Court of Appeals saw it as "unfortunate" but refused to find reversible error on that score.

It noted in passing that since *Durham* was modified by *Mc Donald* in 1962,[4] "insanity acquittals have run at about 2% of all cases terminated" and that within the last seven years "jury verdicts of not guilty by reason of insanity averaged only three per annum."[5] Refusing to regard this as a matter of judicial concern it declared that it "perceived no basis in these data for any conclusion that the number or percentage of insanity acquittals has been either excessive or inadequate."[6]

And thus—in brief—the country's psychiatrically most sophisticated court portrayed the living insanity defense in the Nation's capital with never a doubt that "all's right with the world."

Having reaffirmed for all practical purposes the right of

---

[4] McDonald v. United States, 312 F.2d 847 (D.C. Cir. 1962).
[5] United States v. Brawner, ——F.2d—— (1972).
[6] *Id.*, ——

the St. Elizabeths psychiatric hierarchy to continue its monopoly in deciding the issue of exculpatory mental illness, the Court of Appeals, however, proceeded to repudiate the verbal formulation of *Durham,* ironically on the ground that it furthered a psychiatric usurpation of the determination of criminal responsibility. It saw the "product" test of *Durham* as particularly susceptible to that abuse and recalled the "flip-flop weekend" at St. Elizabeths which resulted in the unexpected declaration that a condition, that is, psychopathy, hitherto not regarded as a disease was thereafter to be regarded as such with a consequent change in the jury verdict.[7] For reasons which appear obscure if not cabalistic, it assumed that the substitution of words more akin to a nineteenth century model for the "product" terminology was more likely to put a damper on such psychiatric usurpation and that a jury would still be able to decide the ultimate issue within a context of wider horizons of knowledge. In *lieu* of the product test of *Durham,* it adopted, with some modification, the twentieth century formulation of *M'Naghten,* sponsored by the conservative *American Law Institute* in its *Model Penal Code* as the key test of criminal responsibility.

The Model Penal Code of the A.L.I. has explicitly sought the inclusion of the so-called psychopath *among the criminally responsible.* To this end, it provides that the terms "mental disease or defect [do] not include an abnormality manifested only by repeated criminal or otherwise anti-social conduct."[8] In a curious attempt at avoiding the charge of judicial formulation of diagnostic criteria while appeasing "conservative" critics of its *Durham* administration, the Court declared that this *caveat* paragraph of the A.L.I. was not to be regarded as part of its new rule, but as "a rule for

[7] Sociopathy, and emotional instability were at one time proclaimed to be conditions rising to the dignity of mental illnesses at St. Elizabeths Hospital—in one case in mid-trial following a weekend conference by the hospital staff. *See* In re Rosenfield, 157 F. Supp. 18 (D.D.C. 1957) *and* Campbell v. United States, 307 F.2d. 597 (D.C. Cir. 1962).

[8] United States v. Brawner, ——F.2d—— (1972).

application by the judge to avoid a miscarriage of justice, not for the inclusion to the jury."

Chief Judge Bazelon concurred, saying that he saw no probable improvement flowing from adoption of a new verbal formula, while noting the continuing problem of the majority of criminal defendants in securing competent psychiatric testimony (presumably outside the ranks of government psychiatrists). He concluded that *Durham* had failed, but declared that "plainly, we did not fail for want of trying."[9]

In a sense, the death certificate issued by the Court of Appeals to its own rule in *Brawner* was well overdue. *Durham* had long ceased to invite testimony as to the "dynamics" of a disease that is, as to "how it occurred, developed and affected the mental and emotional processes of the defendant."[10]

Durham jurisprudence had indeed been defective but above all for a lack of judicial initiative in scrutinizing the credibility of the psychiatric establishment and for lack of a developing procedural apparatus, capable of giving the poor an opportunity to secure the requisite expert testimonial assistance. Yet notwithstanding its failure to give life to such canons of fairness, early *Durham* case law continued to remind decision-makers of their ultimate duty to secure justice, even for those whose poverty had made it impossible for them to secure the type of psychiatric testimony, made available to a John Bradley or a Bernard Goldfine. The total removal of the *Durham* rhetoric from the letter of the law has thus served the function of wiping out a last quivering reminder of essential democratic aspirations, and one is hard put to view this as a matter of small moment. For in scrapping the verbiage of the rule, a rule closely associated in time and spirit with the landmark decision of the Supreme Court in the desegregation of public schools, the Court appeared to be turning the clock back, and in so doing endors-

---

[9] *Id.*——
[10] Carter v. United States, 252 F.2d 608, 617 (D.C. Cir. 1957)

ing a view of life in no way congenial to a fair, comprehensive and scientific assessment of an element of crime conspicuously and irrationally neglected in too many cases—the mental state of the accused. In this context the dominant judicial note seems in line with a "sock it to them" jurisprudence of Nixonian vintage—a jurisprudence in which the burden of proof as to innocence (by virtue of mental disease) has drastically and perhaps unconstitutionally shifted to the defendant[11] and in which the government psychiatrist is subject to *no* scrutiny of his credibility by an appellate court.

HUMAN RIGHTS VIOLATIONS BEFORE BRAWNER

This development of course is not surprising to any moderately independent observer of the District scene. Long before *Brawner* it was clear that the *Durham* rule had ceased to inhibit the irrational and inhumane treatment of the mentally sick offender. Indeed, in inviting testimony to create wider horizons of knowledge in the courtroom, in declaring psychiatric examinations desirable in wider numbers of cases, in "requiring" greater facilities for the poor who relied on exculpatory mental illness as a defense to crime,[12] the *Durham* court appeared to have performed in a manner reminiscent of Macbeth's witches—a promise held to the ear was broken to the hope. Certainly not since 1962 and its accompanying avalanche highlighted by *McDonald* and *Hightower*[13] and the growing hostility of the lower judiciary

---

[11] 24 D.C. Code §301(j) enacted in 1970 (under the impetus of a currently fashionable Law and Order drive)—provides that "no person accused of an offense shall be acquitted on the grounds that he was insane at the time of its commission *unless his insanity is affirmatively established by a preponderance of the evidence.*"

[12] Calloway v. United States, 270 F.2d. 334 (D.C. Cir 1959).
Winn v. United States, 270 F.2d. 326 (D.C. Cir. 1959).

[13] McDonald v. United States, 312 F.2d 847 (D.C. Cir. 1962)
Hightower v. United States, 325 F.2d 616 (D.C. Cir. 1963).

toward the formulation of any insanity defense, remotely reflective of the spirit of 1954—have the District of Columbia courts assured fair, temperate, careful and consistent consideration of the mental condition of defendants who sought to advance an insanity defense even upon the basis of flagrant psychotic symptomatology.

The leeway accorded by the Court of Appeals to District Court interpretations of exculpatory mental illness had moreover been so substantial as to nullify the early promise of *Durham* to seek "wider horizons of knowledge." And as previously noted, the Court of Appeals had refused to interfere with jury verdicts founded on instructions by the trial judge which were couched in the restrictive nineteenth century terminology of M'Naghten.

Nor is it easily forgotten that the recognition by the Court of Appeals of the widest possible spectrum of exculpatory mental illnesses—still under *Durham*—had eroded through affirmances of convictions resting on St. Elizabeths testimony, stating that drug addicts, epileptics, sex perverts and victims of delusionary and hallucinatory experiences were without mental disease or defect.

Civil law countries with more traditional old world views appear to have done better by the defendant. Thus the District of Columbia stands in sharp and disturbing contrast to Norwegian practice which consistently secures the exculpation of the psychotically incapacitated accused—under a rule which holds an act not to be "punishable if committed while the perpetrator was insane or unconscious."[14]

The regression in governing standards of exculpatory mental illness had in fact reached the point where the District

---

[14] Norwegian Penal Code §44, as quoted in J. ANDENAES, THE GENERAL PART OF THE CRIMINAL LAW OF NORWAY (Fred B. Rotterman & Company, 1965) p. 252. The practice emerging under this Norwegian code provision seems to have ensured careful and consistent exclusion of the psychotic patient (and psychosis seems liberally and elastically interpreted in this context) from criminal punishment. Norway has not in this process ex-
(Footnote continued on next page.)

of Columbia was significantly behind jurisdictions upholding more or less enlightened versions of *M'Naghten.*

Brawner thus only hallowed an existing trend. The Court of Appeals spoke of its failure to inquire into psychiatric credibility at a time when the only psychiatrists available to the poor man were those of the government, as expressive of its "unusual deference to the jury on the issue of responsibility."[15] It is obvious, however, that this was in no way expressive of deference to the jury, buffeted as the jury was by a tempestuous prosecutorial appeal to convict in the name of duty, honor, country and a judicial charge expressive of incredulity in the good faith of the insanity defense. It was expressive instead of the most "unusual deference" to the government psychiatrist, elevated as he thus was above all other witnesses in the courtroom.

In this light it was crystal clear long before *Brawner* that it was the government psychiatrist and he alone—acting almost invariably in accord with what he viewed as the government's wishes—who determined the outcome of the case. It is ironic that the *Brawner* court which repudiated *Durham* on the assumption that it tended to depend too heavily on the say-so of psychiatric witnesses should have adopted a doctrine which renders the power of government psychiatrists explicitly and visibly more powerful than ever before. The deference accorded to the testimony of Dr. Platkin was clearly a part of the *Brawner* doctrine—and of far more practical significance than the quasi-medieval theological disquisition resulting in the adoption of the new verbal formula.[16]

---

perienced the problem of psychiatric inhumanity as a consequence of these operations, as we have.

[15] Bazelon, C.J. concurring in United States v. Eichberg, 439 F.2d 620 (D.C. Cir. 1971).

[16] This view appears shared by a psychologist observer of the District scene. "Now . . . the court has adopted a rule which threatens to increase, rather than reduce, the experts' influence over the jury's ultimate decision." Simon, *Brawner Decision: Beyond Science and Determinism,* A.P.A. MONITOR, September-October, 1972.

THE POST-BRAWNER SYNDROME

Durham thus failed to break the critical monopoly of decision-making of a government hospital-prison. (It had not created that monopoly.) *Brawner* now explicitly recognized the propriety of this critical monopoly and announced, however discreetly, that hereafter it would no longer be subject to challenge. The poor of Washington are thus left officially and exclusively dependent upon the graces of the St. Elizabeths staff for the exploration of an insanity defense, and as a consequence of their immunity from scrutiny by an appellate court, St. Elizabeths physicians have acquired a power over the ultimate outcome of a case undiscoverable in the case of any other type of expert witness in the English-speaking world. The government psychiatrist, at least in cases which are overwhelmingly indigent, is, to invert a well-known aphorism, now "on top and not on tap." The continued recognition of his infallibility—from the standpoint of appellate review—makes the doctrine governing *ex cathedra* pronouncements by the Pope seem puny by comparison.[17]

In this light the critical moment of decision-making in the insanity defense would now appear to be not the submission of the case to the jury but the vote taken at a St. Elizabeths staff conference in advance of trial.

One is hard put to discover a pre-1962 situation more inimical to fair and enlightened fact-finding.[18]

---

[17] The private psychiatrist *willing to battle for his patient* against the St. Elizabeths staff has, for all practical purposes, been run out of the courts. A dubious system permitting the haphazard selection of private psychiatrists by the Public Defender Service has enabled isolated individuals to take the field on a pay scale clearly incapable of attracting the best. The batting average of such private psychiatrists against St. Elizabeths is, as described by a member of the Public Defender Service, "about zero." Knowledgeable members of the bar regard the Nixonian courts as effectively devoid of private psychiatrists for the poor.

[18] *Cf.* G. FEIFER, JUSTICE IN MOSCOW, 225-286 (1965).

WHAT WENT WRONG?

In the courts?

Whether lawyer or behavioral scientist, the protagonist of early *Durham* jurisprudence was seen as a disrupting and disturbing element—indistinguishable in any meaningful sense from a member of a subversive group—and he was in fact often treated as such.[19] Sanctions levelled against the lawyer included threats of disbarment and imprisonment. The behavioral scientist fared better but not much better. Intervening years seem to have produced no change in attitudes in this respect.[20] Indeed, it is strikingly characteristic of the precarious status of the insanity defense in the Nation's capital that the *Brawner* case itself was marked by the verbal abuse heaped upon the one psychologist who dared to question a St. Elizabeths judgment attuned to a finding of guilt.

The ease with which pressures can be brought to bear on the unorthodox in no more serious a challenge to the social order than the defense of the drug addict as mentally ill gives rise to serious misgivings as to the ease with which justice can be stampeded on other grounds.

---

[19] The vicissitudes inflicted upon the protagonist of a liberal version of the insanity defense were by no means restricted to the members of the project staff. They were shared by many members of the bar who took the Court of Appeals at its word when it declared (in the early phase of *Durham* jurisprudence) that "the assumption that psychosis is a legally sufficient mental disease and that other illnesses are not is erroneous." The Georgetown Legal Intern Service was a target of very similar attacks in earlier days and has since modified its activities to conform to the expectations of the establishment.

[20] *See* Blunt v. United States, 389 F.2d. 545 (D.C. Cir. 1967).

In the psychiatric establishment?

The consistent failure of the American Psychiatric Association to utter a word in the defense of the drug addict, to say nothing of many a psychotically incapacitated individual in cases litigated in the District of Columbia, or to discipline its membership in a congeries of sleight of hand, raises a serious question concerning the integrity of American psychiatry *in toto,* at least insofar as it is represented by its parent organization. Any doubts concerning the political orientation of the American Psychiatric Association would seem resolved by its *amicus* brief, urging adoption of the A.L.I. version of *M'Naghten* in the *Brawner* case. The motivation of this action would seem transparent. *Durham* jurisprudence had catapulted too many private psychiatrists in opposition to the verdict of government psychiatry into the courtroom arena, and if the ensuing spectacle had not been flattering to the psychiatric profession, then indeed any standard—however obsolete—which would seem less destructive to the pocketbooks and reputations of the profession would seem preferable.

SOME LESSONS FROM DURHAM IN THE DISTRICT OF COLUMBIA

What does *Durham* have to teach those who seek more equitable and rational reconsideration of the insanity defense in other jurisdictions?

First and foremost, and the lesson is obvious, *Durham* points to the substantial irrelevance of the verbal formulation of a test of criminal responsibility. This of course in no way discounts the significance of the symbolism of the test, a symbolism capable of suggesting the propriety or the impropriety of a rational and compassionate concern for the ordeal of the mentally disordered offender. Seen in this light, the extinction of the symbolism of *Durham* is a disaster second only to that of its maladministration. *But aside from the symbolism,* operations under Durham—as indeed under any other rule—are shaped by available material and intellectual resources and a willingness by the relevant decision-makers to proceed in accord with expanding horizons of knowledge. Certainly at present such a willingness seems diminutive.

The exquisite sensitivity of the body politic to any measure reflective of a change in traditional rules of criminal responsibility points, for the present at least, to the limited effectiveness of judicial activism in initiating and sustaining social change in this field, if only in the District of Columbia. Must effective reform hinge at all times on the initiation of new policy by the legislature?

More important, however, than the enunciation of new policy through legal doctrine, is the development of new human and material resources designed to make the enunciation of policy more than mere empty rhetoric. The most forward-looking doctrine of exculpatory mental illness will founder upon the reefs of inadequate psychiatric facilities, materially and intellectually impoverished hospitals, and the hostility of a significant segment of the public—including much of the psychiatric and judicial professions.[21]

---

[21] The matter has been exhaustively and imaginatively explored by the late Professor George H. Dession. See Dession, *Psychiatry and the Conditioning of Criminal Justice,* 47 YALE L. J. 319 (1947). Professor Hermann Mannheim aptly described some of Professor Dession's concern in these words:

"Individualization of criminal justice? Certainly—but can it be so conditioned as to avoid the dangers associated in our minds with the *lettres de cachet* of French prerevolutionary times and similar devices also adopted under the slogan of individualized justice? And is individualization, to the extent implied in an application of psychiatry that would be more than mere lip-service, not something entirely beyond the means available for the purpose? It is the ever widening discrepancy between the standard modern society expects and the burden it is willing to shoulder that worried Dession as it worried some other observers who, although sincerely in favor of the Welfare State realize that some of its demands are far removed from practical politics."

H. Mannheim, *George H. Dession,* 5 BUFFALO L. REV. 9, 10 (1955).

Certainly there would seem little hope for constructive change until the appearance of more psychiatrists, more skilled and more appropriately committed to the ideology of a democratic social order and more judges prepared to hear before they condemn.[22]

ABOLISH THE INSANITY DEFENSE? WHY NOT!

A simplistic solution and the one endorsed by psychiatric stalwarts like Karl Menninger, is the abolition of the insanity defense. Dr. Menninger suggests that a psychiatric diagnostic center take over the task of "rehabilitation" after the conviction of the accused.[23] With what one knows of the existing horrors of psychiatric administration, carried out in the light of day and often in the courtroom, one shudders at the operations to be expected of the psychiatric Star Chamber—screened from all manner of public scrutiny and focusing upon an individual stripped of his rights—devoid of the presumption of innocence—and sequestered in a bastille—which whether run by psychiatric or conventional jailers—has not ceased to be the most clearly perceptible bastion of tyranny in our social order.

---

[22] The true pitfalls of the current legal psychiatric scene will have to be faced before reforms are possible. What is called for as a first step is more hard-headed reporting as to the realities of psychiatric and judicial decision-making in the most elementary political sense of who gets what, when and how. The abandonment of the fatuous preoccupation with alleged problems of communication between lawyers and psychiatrists, a preoccupation which serves more to obscure than to reveal—so typical of almost all the academic writing at this time—is well overdue. For to this day the legally unskilled journalist has remained the only source of credible and valid information as to hospitals and courts, essential to the rational consideration of legal reform. *See*, e.g. A. DEUTSCH, THE SHAME OF THE STATES (1948); J. MITFORD, THE TRIAL OF DR. SPOCK, THE REVEREND WILLIAM SLOANE COFFIN JR., MICHAEL FERBER, MICHAEL GOODMAN AND MARKUS RASKIN (1969).

[23] K. MENNINGER, THE CRIME OF PUNISHMENT (1968).

Outright repeal of the insanity defense, extending to the exclusion of the psychiatric profession from the pre-conviction stage, conjures up such episodes of a not so ancient past as those in which judges ordered the whipping of a church bell for a failure to ring out an alarm against an attempted assassination of a member of the Royal Family in Czarist Russia, or the hanging of a pig which had attacked a child as a warning to like-minded malefactors—all a little over a hundred years ago. Concern for the mental element of "crime" is, after all, relatively recent—but it is clearly a touchstone of the civilizing quality of our law. And it is this very quality which has been put in jeopardy in the District of Columbia and beyond it.

The new abolitionists invoke the spirit of liberty. They do so, however, under circumstances painfully reminiscent of the adage that some of the greatest crimes are committed in its name.

Inevitably the abolitionist proposal will meet with almost uniform revulsion on the part of any lawyer conversant with criminal practice and committed to the ideology of the Bill of Rights. Such a lawyer will have met too many clients manifesting the suffering experienced by the "mentally or emotionally ill" to regard their condition as a mere "myth of mental illness." He will have seen too much of the brutality of the prison system to wish to abandon any man or woman, entrusted to his charge, to its torments—least of all one already so gravely handicapped as the "mentally ill." To him, there is nothing mythical about the suffering of a James Rivers or a Walter Wilson and the suggestion that he regard it as "myth" in line with some currently fashionable claptrap strikes him as more appropriate to the administration of the garrison-prison state than to that of the free society. Such a lawyer will not be unaware of the fact that hospitals have indeed been often transformed into prisons and he will not rest content until such hospitals are hospitals in fact as well as name and until coercive confinement in such hospitals does comply with procedures consistent with due process.[24] That, of course, was the very purpose of the exercise in the Lynch case.

He will feel strongly that rational reform cannot involve yet another commitment to a prison system which has been found bankrupt at every significant level.[25] However horrendous present psychiatric practices, he will see them, unlike prison practices, as generally open to public scrutiny and hence—notwithstanding the alarums and flourishes of the establishment—as subject to some measure of corrective change. (The pace of such change is, of course, directly proportioned to appropriately politicized demand.) He will see no comparable situation in the context of the prison system. He will know from his experience as defense counsel that the prison system is effectively screened by an iron curtain save for rare occasions; that at its best its commitment is symbolized in the Quaker motto of "Labor, Silence, Penitence"; and that at its worst, it permits the massacre of prisoners recently encountered in the State of Arkansas.[26]

Finally, such a lawyer, and I like to think that he represents a not insignificant segment of the American Bar,

---

[24] For an imaginative, humane and carefully conceived program designed to secure the continuing protection of patient rights—after an insanity acquittal see 112 Cong. Rec., (No. 127) August 4, 1966 (Senator Robert F. Kennedy's introductory discussion of his bill to provide treatment of persons acquitted on the ground of insanity.

[25] Brutality, widespread recidivism and few rehabilitative results are disclosed as characteristic of the prison system in most scientific surveys. For a summary of some contemporary data see R. ARENS AND H.D. LASSWELL, IN DEFENSE OF PUBLIC ORDER, 96, 100 (1961).

[26] "The Arkansas State Police began an investigation today after penitentiary officials recovered three skeletons from an unmarked burial ground on the Cummins State Prison Farm and suggested that scores of others might be found there. Gov. Winthrop Rockefeller, a Republican, said at a news conference in Little Rock today that yesterday's discovery of the skeletons was 'shocking.' He promised that the police would explore 'the whole question.' 'I don't think there's any question that some of the bodies that will be found may show signs of violent death,' the Governor said. A prison official estimated that the remains of as many as 300 others might be buried at the prison." New York Times, January 31, 1968, at p. 17.

will view the insanity defense (and ultimately a better name will be substituted for this elementary procedural safeguard for the accused in a legal system dedicated to the preservation of human dignity) as a defense calculated to produce reasoned and compassionate inquiry.

He will think of *Durham* as a well-motivated reform which failed and he will feel that this failure must be understood if we are to do better in the future. He will recall moreover, that, turned upon the living scene of courts and hospitals, *Durham* did *more* than state a pious principle: it threw into bold relief the discrepancies between aspiration and performance; it rendered visible the continuing plight of the mentally ill and, above all, the impoverished mentally ill in our system of criminal justice; it revealed for all to see "the monstrous practice of punishing a product of illness," a practice it did not significantly inhibit; it experienced its own frailty—and in this process the frailty of the rule of law against powerful and entrenched interests.

For all the horrors of its maladministration, *Durham* remained to many a symbol of hope for a better and gentler day—a hope now emphatically denied by *Brawner*, Bazelon, C.J., concurring.

The *judicially* sponsored experiment calculated to enhance the rights of the accused under *Durham* has thus come to an end with *Brawner*—with its accompanying lament by the ever present Judge Bazelon—"not with a bang but a whimper." The upward road toward a civilized code of correction will have to be traveled anew.

Much has been learned in encounters with organized resistance to change in the interim. Further steps to minimize much of what remains of savagery in our law remain overdue. It is safe to predict that the "whimper" of *Brawner* is far from the last sound in this strange eventful history.

APPENDIX I

COMPTROLLER GENERAL OF THE UNITED STATES

WASHINGTON 25

B-150346   June 10, 1963

Dear Mr. Secretary:

Reference is made to our letter of November 29, 1962, and enclosure, to you, requesting a report concerning Federal grant funds allocated by the National Institutes of Health to the Washington School of Psychiatry together with your views on the propriety of using such grant funds to pay expert witnesses testifying for a defendant in a criminal case, and your reply thereto, dated March 28, 1963. Enclosed with your letter was a report in the matter prepared by the Public Health Service and a copy of a memorandum from your General Counsel to the Surgeon General, Public Health Service.

Our request for your views in this matter resulted from information we received indicating that in the trial of the case of *United States* v. *Willie Lee Stewart* (held in the United States District Court for the District of Columbia) Federal grant funds were used by the Washington School of Psychiatry to pay expert witnesses (one psychologist and six psychiatrists) for examining the defendant in the above-cited case and also for testifying in court on his behalf. The information we received further disclosed that the defendant, on motion of his counsel, was examined at Saint Elizabeths Hospital by staff of the Hospital and found without mental defect or mental disease. The report prepared by the Public Health Service discloses that in April 1961, a grant, Research Project No. M-5009, was awarded by the National Institute of Mental Health to the Washington School of Psychiatry. The report discloses that psychiatrists serving as expert witnesses in cases involving indigent defendants in criminal cases have received compensation totaling $1,970 from the funds awarded under this grant.

It is stated in the report that the particular purpose of this grant or project was to conduct research on the problem of the defense of insanity within the District of Columbia and its significance for the general problem of criminal law and psychiatry. It is further stated that this study was designed to uncover and weigh variables involved in the key decisions leading to the determination of criminal responsibility when an insanity defense is interposed in a criminal trial and thus shed light upon operative legal psychiatric concepts of insanity.

. . . .

It is stated in the report that the methods of data collection . . . include . . . the use of personal interviews, . . . content analysis of judicial instructions to the jury . . . examination and analysis of abstracted cases and the trial of actual cases within the context of which all the variables referred to earlier would be examined *in vivo,* so to speak. We are advised that it was in the course of these test cases that the grant funds were utilized to pay psychiatric witnesses, since this was felt to be an essential portion of the research project. The report discloses that the research project in question was approved by the Surgeon General under the broad authority vested in him by section 301 of the Public Health Service Act, approved July 1, 1944, ch. 373, 58 Stat. 691, as amended 42 U.S.C. 241.

The Public Health Service report states in conclusion that inasmuch as the use of expert witnesses constitutes an essential element in the successful conduct of this project, and since the investigator, in his application, clearly indicated his intention to use grant funds for this purpose, it is their view that the expenditure of grant funds for the provision of psychiatric witnesses on behalf of defendants in criminal cases within the context of the project involved was appropriate and that no question of propriety is involved.

Your General Counsel in his memorandum to the Surgeon General states that the Public Health Service report presents a persuasive case for the propriety of the expenditures in question, in terms of the research objective and the availability of funds. However, the General Counsel further states that he is seriously troubled by the impropriety of conducting research in the courtroom without the knowledge and approval of the court, when the research involves participation in the processes of a trial.[1] In the memorandum the General Counsel advised the Surgeon General as follows:

"The Secretary has asked me to request you take steps to assure that in the future no such practice is supported by the Public Health Service in the conduct of this or other projects."

Section 301 of the Public Health Service Act, as amended, provides, in part, as follows:

"The Surgeon General shall conduct in the Service and encourage, cooperate with, and render assistance to other appropriate public authorities, scientific institutions, and scientists in the conduct of, and promote the coordination of, research, investigations, experiments, demonstrations, and studies relating to the causes, diagnosis, treatment, control, and prevention of physical and mental diseases and impairments of man. . . . In carrying out the foregoing the Surgeon General is authorized to—

 . . . .

"Make grants-in-aid to universities, hospitals, laboratories, and other public or private institutions, and to individuals

---

[1] In point of fact—the Comptroller General's report appears to have been at least partially in error. The Chief Judge of the U.S. Court of Appeals, was explicitly informed of project operations. (my footnote)

for such research projects as are recommended by . . . or, with respect to mental health, recommended by the National Advisory Mental Health Council. . . ."

While the authority vested in the Surgeon General by the above-quoted provision of law is very broad, we have serious doubts that the Congress contemplated or intended, in connection with research relating to mental diseases, that Federal grant funds be used to pay expert witnesses (psychiatrists or psychologists) to testify on behalf of defendants, indigent or otherwise, in a criminal trial. In this connection we might point out here, that as far as Federal District Courts are concerned provision is specifically made in Rule 17(b), Federal Rules of Criminal Procedure, page 3419, Title 18, United States Code, for attendance of witnesses in the case of indigent defendants. See also Rule 28 of the same Rules, page 3425, Title 18, United States Code.

Further, there would appear to be little difference in using Federal grant funds, such as are involved here, to pay the fees of expert psychiatric witnesses in a case where the defense of insanity is involved and using such funds to pay the defendant's attorney in the same case. We doubt that anyone would seriously contend that it would be proper in such circumstances to use Federal grant funds to pay the defendant's attorney. While it may be proper in connection with research into the problem of the defense of insanity to use Federal grant funds in connection with the cost of psychiatric examination of defendants in criminal cases whose sanity appears questionable, it does not follow that such funds are also available to pay the persons conducting such examinations for testifying in court, on behalf of such defendants.

In light of the foregoing as well as for the reason set forth in your General Counsel's memorandum it is our view that funds granted pursuant to the authority contained in section 301 of the Public Health Service Act, as amended, may not be used to pay expert psychiatric witnesses to testify on behalf of a defendant in a criminal case. However, inasmuch as the expenditures involved in the instant case apparently were made in good faith and since pursuant to your direction steps are to be taken by the Public Health Service to insure that in the future Federal grant funds will not be used for such purpose, we will take no further action in the matter.

Sincerely yours,
Joseph Campbell
Comptroller General
of the United States

The Honorable
The Secretary of Health, Education, and Welfare

APPENDIX II

The following is illustrative material as to jury charges in the District of Columbia between 1960 and 1962. The materials have been culled from three jury charges by three different judges and are designed to provide a preliminary impression of the problems raised by judicial instructions governing the insanity defense. In Case No. 1, the jury was charged *inter alia* as follows:

> The only question to be determined by you is whether he has committed the offense with which he is charged and whether he should be held responsible for it. Everything else is extraneous and must be set to one side.
>
> I shall commence my discussion of the law by summarizing a few general principles that are applicable to all criminal cases, including, of course, this one.
>
> First, the fact that a defendant has been indicted and is charged with a crime is not in itself to be taken as an indication of guilt because an indictment is merely the procedure and the machinery by which a defendant is brought before the court and is placed on trial.
>
> Second, every defendant in a criminal case is presumed to be innocent and this presumption of innocence attaches to the defendant throughout the trial until it is overcome by evidence. That is one of the basic principles of our criminal law.
>
> Third, the burden of proof is on the government to prove the defendant's guilt beyond a reasonable doubt. Unless the government sustains this burden and proves beyond a reasonable doubt that the defendant has committed every element of the offense with which he is charged and should be held responsible for it, the jury must find him not guilty. Now let me repeat. The burden of proof on the government is to establish the defendant's guilt beyond a reasonable doubt and not necessarily beyond all doubt whatsoever.
>
> Proof beyond a reasonable doubt may be defined as proof to a moral certainty and not necessarily proof to an absolute or mathematical certainty. By a reasonable doubt, as its very name

implies, is meant a doubt based on reason and not just some whimsical speculation or some capricious conjecture.

I think I can explain to you, ladies and gentlemen, the meaning of the words proof beyond a reasonable doubt in simple everyday language. Proof beyond a reasonable doubt does not mean that the evidence has to be all one way. Proof beyond a reasonable doubt simply means this: If after an impartial comparison and consideration of all the evidence on one side and on the other you can say to yourself that you are not satisfied of the defendant's guilt or his responsibility, then you have a reasonable doubt. But, on the other hand, if after such impartial comparison and consideration of all the evidence on both sides you can truthfully and candidly say to yourself that you have an abiding conviction of the defendant's guilt and his responsibility, such as you would be willing to act upon in the more weighty and important matters relating to your own affairs, then you have no reasonable doubt.

In other words, to summarize, proof beyond a reasonable doubt is such proof as will result in an abiding conviction of the defendant's guilt on your part, such a conviction as you would be willing to act upon in the more weighty and important matters relating to your own affairs.

In determining whether the government has established the charge against the defendant beyond a reasonable doubt as well as his responsibility, you will consider and weigh the testimony of all the witnesses who have testified at this trial, as well as all the circumstances concerning which testimony has been introduced. Circumstances frequently cast an illuminating light on oral testimony.

You are the sole judges of the credibility of witnesses, the law says. That means that it is for you and for you alone to determine whether to believe any witness, the extent to which any witnesses should be credited and the weight to be attached to the testimony of any witness. On those issues as to which there is any conflict in the testimony it is your function to resolve the conflict and to determine where the truth lies and what the fact was.

. . . .

The defendant, as has been said all along, is charged with violations of the law relating to narcotics. Narcotics have a recognized legitimate use in medicine. On the other hand, their use when not under the supervision of a physician is regarded as dangerous and as susceptible of an evil influence. Consequently, the law has to regulate traffic in narcotics in such a way as to make them available for medicinal purposes under the supervision of a physician, but at the same time to suppress them when they are attempted to be used for illicit and illegitimate uses. Consequently, the law prescribes certain limitations, which I shall discuss in a moment, on the method in which narcotics are handled.

The law relating to narcotic drugs applies to opium, cocoa

leaves, opiate, and any compound, salt, derivative or preparation thereof. The Government chemist testified that heroin hydrochloride, which is the narcotic drug involved in this case, is a derivative of opium. Consequently, the law relating to narcotics applies to heroin hydrochloride.

The specific charge against the defendant is that on October 19th, 1961, he sold nine capsules to Agent Herman H. Scott of the Federal Bureau of Narcotics, the capsules containing heroin hydrochloride; Agent Scott, of course, at that time working under cover and the fact that he was a government agent not being known to the defendant.

. . . .
. . . . The defendant, . . . , interposes what is known as a defense of insanity. It is not strictly a defense. He raises, more accurately, the issue of insanity.

In a case in which the defendant's sanity is in issue, that is, if some evidence is introduced creating a reasonable doubt concerning the defendant's mental responsibility, then the government has a two-fold burden of proof. First, as has been indicated to you by me, the government must prove beyond a reasonable doubt that the defendant committed the crime charged in the indictment. Second, and in addition, the government must prove beyond a reasonable doubt that the defendant was mentally responsible for the crime with which he is charged, and I shall expand what is meant by mental responsibility in a moment or two.

If it is not established beyond a reasonable doubt that the defendant committed the crime with which he is charged, of course your verdict would be not guilty. If, however, it is established that the defendant committed the crime, but it is not established beyond a reasonable doubt that he was mentally responsible for the crime, then the jury must find him not guilty on the ground of insanity, and you must expressly specify not guilty on the ground of insanity because if you find him not guilty on the ground of insanity the law requires the court, and the court has no alternative, immediately to commit the defendant to a mental hospital, and the defendant would not be released from such mental hospital unless and until the superintendent of that hospital certifies to the court that the defendant has recovered his sanity, that in the opinion of the superintendent the defendant will not in the reasonable future be dangerous to himself or others, and that in the opinion of the superintendent the defendant is entitled to his unconditional release from the hospital.

Upon the receipt of such a certificate the court decides, with or without a hearing, whether the defendant may be unconditionally released from the hospital, and in order that he may be released the court must find that the defendant has recovered his sanity and will not in the reasonable future be dangerous to himself or others.

Now to discuss the question of mental responsibility in somewhat greater detail. It is claimed in behalf of the defendant that he should not be held responsible for the offense with which he is charged on the alleged ground that at the time the offense was committed by him, if it was committed by him, he was suffering from a mental disease and the offense was the product of the mental disease.

Indeed, in certain instances the law does not hold an insane person responsible for his acts or a mentally defective person. In order to be responsible for his acts a person must have the mental capacity to commit the act with which he is charged.

It is not, however, in every case in which the accused is suffering from some mental abnormality or some mental deficiency or defect or from some mental disorder that he is to be deemed free from liability for his crimes and not responsible for his acts. There are many abnormal persons or many persons with mental deficiencies or persons suffering from personality disorders or mental disorders whom the law holds responsible, in certain instances, for crimes that such persons may commit. Obviously, there are good reasons for this.

On the other hand, there are certain types of persons afflicted with mental disease or mental defects who are not held responsible for particular crimes. The law on this point is this: that if the defendant was suffering from some mental disease or from some mental defect, that is, if he had a diseased or defective mental condition at the time when the crime was committed, and, further —and this is very important—if the crime itself was the product of that mental disease or defect, then and only then the defendant is not responsible for his criminal act.

Now, then, what is a mental disease? In this instance, as I understand it, it is not claimed that the defendant has a mental defect, but that he had a mental disease. A mental disease or defect, the law says, is any abnormal condition of mind which substantially affects mental or emotional processes and substantially impairs behavior control.

Consequently, if you should be convinced beyond a reasonable doubt either that the defendant was not suffering from a mental disease or mental defect, or even if he were so suffering at the time he committed the crime, the crime was not the product or result of the mental disease or mental defect, you may find the defendant guilty, assuming, of course that you find that the fact of the crime is properly established.

Every person is presumed to be sane until the contrary appears. This presumption is founded on human experience. This presumption, however, does not mean that the burden of proof is on the defendant to prove insanity. In cases in which sanity is properly in issue the burden is on the government, on the issue of insanity or mental capacity, just as it is on every other issue, and that burden must be sustained beyond a reasonable doubt. In other words, the government must disprove what we may loosely call the defense of insanity—it is not technically a defense, but what we might call the defense of insanity—beyond a reasonable doubt.

Now, I have already explained to you what a reasonable doubt means. Proof beyond a reasonable doubt does not mean that the evidence must be all one way. It does not mean proof beyond all doubt whatsoever. It means proof to a moral certainty and not to a mathematical or absolute certainty. I shall not repeat the rather extensive definition of proof beyond a reasonable doubt that I gave you earlier in my remarks.

In considering the defense of insanity you have a right to consider whether the defendant knew the difference between right and wrong, whether he acted under the compulsion of an irresistible impulse or had been deprived of or lost the power of his will. You are not, however, limited to considering these matters, but you may consider all of the evidence, lay evidence and expert evidence, in order to reach a conclusion, first whether the defendant was or was not suffering from a mental disease or defect, and, second, if he was, whether the crime was the product of that mental disease.

If you find that the defendant was not suffering from a mental disease or defect at the time of the commission of the offense, then, of course, you may not find him not guilty on the ground of insanity. But even if you find that he was suffering from a mental disease or mental defect, that is not sufficient to justify a verdict of not guilty on the ground of insanity. Then the question arises whether the crime was produced by his mental disease. Consequently, if you reach the conclusion that the crime was *not produced by his mental disease,* even if he had one, then, too, you may not find him not guilty on the ground of insanity. Obviously, even an insane person may at times do things that are entirely rational in and of themselves and that have no connection with his mental disease.

Now let me summarize briefly the evidence on both sides on the issue of mental capacity, and again I repeat what I said earlier, that what I say about the evidence is intended only to help you. You are not bound by my discussion of the evidence. You must reach your own decision on the facts and on the evidence. That, I repeat, is your function, your duty and your responsibility.

The defendant called two psychiatrists—well, before I take that up, the government, anticipating that the question would be raised, called Agent Thompson as a witness, Agent Thompson of the Narcotics Bureau, and he testified that after the defendant was arrested he talked with the defendant at No. 1 Precinct; that he detected no abnormality in him; the defendant's answers were clear and responsive, he appeared to be in full control of his senses and appeared to be normal mentally.

Now, the law admits testimony of a lay observer, of a lay

witness, on the question of mental capacity, just as it does the testimony of an expert witness, and both must be considered by the jury.

The defendant then called two psychiatrists. The first of the psychiatrists was Dr. Hamman and he expressed the opinion that on the date on which this offense is charged to have been committed the defendant was suffering from what is known in the science of psychiatry as a schizoid personality, which the doctor said was a mental disease. He also expressed the opinion that, in his view, the crime said to have been committed by the defendant was the product of his mental illness but he qualified his answer. He said it was the product of his mental illness if the defendant sold narcotics solely in order to be able to get some for himself, but, on the other hand, if he sold narcotics as an ordinary transaction, then it would not be the product of the mental illness. Dr. Hamman also admitted that the defendant's illness, in his opinion, did not affect his ability to distinguish right from wrong. He testified on cross examination that the defendant had an IQ, as it is called, of 95; namely, that he had a normal intellect. He also expressed the opinion that at the moment he sold the nine capsules to Agent Scott he, the defendant, was not moved by an irresistible impulse. He further admitted that at the staff conference in St. Elizabeths Hospital, at which the defendant was questioned, the defendant acted and responded in a normal manner, that he had no delusions, no hallucinations, and that during the three months he was at the hospital there was no wild hysteria. As I recall it, Dr. Hamman testified that in his opinion the schizoid personality, this mental illness with which the defendant has been afflicted, has existed for something like twenty-five or more years.

Now, the next psychiatrist called by the defense was Dr. Legler. Dr. Legler was a young psychiatrist who had just finished his training last June and received his first appointment as a psychiatrist last July as a member of the staff of St. Elizabeths Hospital. He also expressed the opinion that the defendant has a schizoid personality, which is a mental disease, that in his opinion the condition has existed for anywhere from twenty-nine to thirty-two years, and that the crime with which he is charged was the product of mental disease. He expressed the opinion that the defendant's behavior controls were impaired, but not entirely obliterated.

The defendant also called a lay witness, the defendant's wife, Edna Jackson. She testified that he was a moody type of person; but she could not say, she said, whether the defendant was of sound or unsound mind.

Now, the government then called Dr. David J. Owens. Dr. Owens is the Clinical Director of the Maximum Security Division of St. Elizabeths Hospital. He is the chief of that division and he is the superior officer of Dr. Legler and Dr. Hamman, Dr.

Hamman and Dr. Legler being under him. Dr. Owens testified that the defendant had no mental disease, that he had no symptoms of schizoid personality. He was questioned closely on cross-examination as to why and how he came to the conclusion the defendant had no mental disease. His answer was that he found no symptoms of mental disease. He expressed the opinion that drug addiction, without other symptoms, is not a mental disease; at times it may be the result of mental illness, but it is not, according to Dr. Owens, in and of itself a mental disease. He also expressed the opinion that while at the hospital the defendant was in good contact with his surroundings, he was coherent and showed no symptoms of mental disease whatever, and that in his particular case the drug addiction was not related to any mental disease whatever.

Now, the question whether the defendant at the time of the commission of the crime with which he is charged was suffering from a mental disease is for the jury to determine. The decision of the jury cannot be controlled by expert opinions on either side. The jury must determine for itself, from all of the testimony, lay testimony and expert testimony whether a mental disease or defect existed; and, if so, whether the crime was the product of that condition. After all, trial by jury under our law requires a decision by the jurors and not a decision by the experts on either side." U.S. v. Francis E. Jackson, Crim. No. 382-62, given on October 15, 1962, Official Transcript of Proceedings, at 2-23.

In Case No. 2, the jury was charged *inter alia* as follows:

> . . . being fact finders, judges of the facts, you are to approach your task and perform your task objectively, detachedly, and unemotionally. You are not to let sympathy or prejudice or bias or emotion of any kind enter into your thinking, into your deliberations, or into your verdict.
> Now, there have been five witnesses called who are known in the law as expert witnesses; namely, Dr. Ryan, Dr. Platkin, Dr. Owens, Dr. Dobbs, and one other, the neurosurgeon, Dr. Green. All but Dr. Green are psychiatrists. Dr. Green is a neurosurgeon or neurologist and not a psychiatrist. The psychiatrists have testified in relation to the mental condition of the defendant. Dr. Green, of course, being a neurologist, was not qualified on that point as an expert.
> . . . .
> Now a person who by education or experience becomes well versed in a science such as psychiatry, which is a branch of medicine, is permitted to give testimony in respect of that science if it is material to the case.
> In this case insanity is a defense, and the psychiatrists are

specialists who have been called to express their opinions in relation to defendant's mental condition. In weighing their testimony, you will take into consideration their experience and training, the opportunity they had to form an opinion, the reasons given by them for their opinion in determining how much weight you will give to the opinion of each of the psychiatrists who have testified. You will also apply the same criterion to Dr. Green's testimony when you weigh his testimony in respect to his specialty.

Now, of course, in connection with this defense of insanity, you should consider the testimony of the lay witnesses. They are not excluded as bearing on this question.

Now this defendant enters the case as all defendants clothed with the presumption of innocence. That presumption abides with him throughout the trial until it has been overcome by evidence which convinces you of guilt beyond a reasonable doubt. The burden of proof rests upon the government to establish its case beyond a reasonable doubt.

Now, what is a reasonable doubt? A reasonable doubt is such a doubt as would cause a juror after careful and candid consideration and comparison of the evidence to be so undecided that he cannot say he has an abiding conviction of the defendant's guilt. It is such a doubt as would cause a juror to hesitate or pause in the graver or more important transactions of life. However, it is not a whimsical doubt nor a fanciful doubt nor a doubt based on groundless conjecture. It is a doubt for which you can give a reason. The government is not required to establish guilt to a mathematical certainty or a scientific certainty or beyond all doubt. Its burden is to establish guilt beyond a reasonable doubt.

Now when you go to the jury room, you will take with you the indictment. The indictment is not evidence. It is simply a statement of the charges which have been made against this defendant by the grand jury after hearing one side of the case only.

Now the indictment in this case is in ten counts. Each count is in effect a separate charge, and you will be required to reach your verdict on each count separately and render your verdict on each count separately.

The first count charges housebreaking. The second count charges petty larceny. The third, fifth, seventh, and ninth counts charge the offense of forgery. The fourth, sixth, eighth, and tenth counts charge the offense of uttering a forged check.

Now the defense in this case is insanity, but that does not relieve you of the responsibility of determining whether or not the government has established that the defendant committed the acts charged against him in each of the counts in this indictment. If you find that the government has not as to any or all of these counts, your verdict will be not guilty on such count or counts; and that will end the matter in respect to such count or counts. If you find that it has, you will pass on to the question of insanity.

. . . .

When a man is put to trial on a criminal charge, his sanity is presumed; and, therefore, the government does not ordinarily have to introduce evidence on the subject. When, however, as in this case, the issue of defendant's insanity is raised by the introduction of evidence to that effect, this presumption disappears and has no evidentiary weight; and the government has the burden of proving beyond a reasonable doubt that the defendant was mentally responsible for his acts on the dates charged in the various counts of the indictment; that is, February 6, 1961, February 14, 1961, Fabruary 24, 1961, March 10, 1961, and March 16, 1961. These are the crucial dates.

Evidence has been admitted as to his mental condition on these dates and on other dates, but this latter only for the purpose of enabling you to consider that evidence to determine his condition as to the dates of the alleged crime.

You have heard the testimony of the psychiatrists who have taken the stand and also the testimony of the other witnesses who have testified as to his mental condition and also the portions of the D.C. General Hospital records and the Saint Elizabeths Hospital records which have been read to you; and I shall briefly review some of that testimony.

Now these psychiatrists have differed in their opinion. You may consider some of their opinions unclear and uncertain. However, medicine is not an exact science, and this is particularly true of psychiatry; but you will have to weigh and evaluate those opinions and find the truth as best you can, it being the policy of the law that a person mentally irresponsible for his criminal acts should not be punished; but, on the other hand, it is equally the policy of the law that a person should not escape punishment if he is mentally responsible.

Now the defendant has called as witnesses on this issue of defendant's insanity the defendant's wife, the director of the school, Mr. Janson, Mrs. Gallivan, his supervisor at the Mayflower, Dr. Ryan, Dr. Dobbs, and Dr. Green. He has also offered in evidence portions of the records of the D. C. General Hospital while he was a patient there in the spring of 1960.

Briefly, Mr. Janson testified that the defendant during his attendance at the school from March 2, 1959, to February 3, 1960, and from April 18, 1960, and for about ten days thereafter, was withdrawn and solemn and not approachable, although he worked on his drawings and was an average student and knew what he was doing. Also, that he was quiet and reserved and nervous. That covers the period from March 1959 to April 1960.

The defendant's wife testified as to numerous incidents before and after he was a patient at D.C. General Hospital in 1960 during which time the defendant had epileptic seizures on numerous occasions and conducted himself irrationally, was confused and had hallucinations and delusions. I shall not recount all of them, but I do recall she testified that on occasion he fell flat on the ground, ran out in the snow without a coat, prayed in the snow, ran out of the church after going forward to become a member, referred to God and his mother talking to him when his mother was dead, believing the Russians were going to bomb us, put cereal and sugar on the floor, and broke off parts of plants and arranged them on the furniture, tore up the marriage certificate and left his wife, and then later on during the nighttime threw stones at her house and rang her bell and threatened her and was generally violent and belligerent.

Briefly the hospital records as offered in evidence disclose delusions and hallucinations of somewhat the same character, as well as numerous epileptic seizures.

Briefly, his supervisor at the Mayflower, Mrs. Gallivan, testified that before he went to D. C. General Hospital he was a good worker, neat, got along well with other members of the hotel staff and with the guests. After his experience in the hospital when he came back in April of 1960, he was belligerent and had similar delusions and hallucinations to the effect that God was in personal contact with him and gave him certain instructions, a belief that some of the guests were Russian spies, and generally that the defendant was unable to get along with the other members of the staff or the guests and believed that everyone was against him.

The defendant has also offered the testimony of Dr. Ryan who has given his opinion that the defendant on the critical dates in question was suffering from a mental disease, namely, chronic paranoid schizophrenia, and that this disease caused him to commit the acts charged in the indictment, or that the acts if committed by him were the product of this mental disease. Dr. Ryan also testified that the defendant was incapable of *distinguishing between right and wrong* because of his mental disease, and that may be considered by you as bearing upon whether or not the acts, if committed by him, were the *product of this mental disease*. Dr. Ryan has gone very fully into the reasons and basis for his opinion.

Now the government, on the other hand, has called a number of witnesses as to what took place at the time of the alleged forgeries and uttering, and has offered the officer's testimony as to what the defendant said when he was arrested and what he put in writing at the time of his arrest and contends that the manner of entering the school, the kind of checks which were taken, namely, payroll checks, the taking of the identification card of another person and putting his own photograph on that card, and the manner in which the checks were cashed and the method used by the defendant in establishing his identity in order to cash the checks, his attitude and demeanor at the time of his arrest, show a purposeful planning, scheming, and rational mind. The government has also called Dr. Platkin of the psychiatric staff of Saint Elizabeths and Dr. Owens of the same staff who testified that in their opinion the defendant was free of any mental disease or defect at the time of the offenses alleged in the indictment were committed. They likewise have gone very fully into the reasons and basis for their opinions.

. . . .

Now, it will be your duty to weigh all this relevant evidence and determine whether the government has established beyond a reasonable doubt that the defendant was not suffering from a mental disease or defect at the time in question, or that the act was not the product of such diseases or defect if one existed.

Unless you believe beyond a reasonable doubt that he was not suffering from a mental disease or defect or if he was that the criminal acts charged against him were not the product of such disease or defect, you must find the defendant not guilty by reason of insanity, notwithstanding your conclusion of guilt on one or more of the counts in this indictment.

Thus your task will not be completed upon finding that the defendant suffered from a mental disease or defect. He would still be guilty of these unlawful acts if he committed them if there was no causal connection between such mental abnormality and the acts.

Now, I have used the term disease. I use it in the sense of a condition which is either capable of improving or deteriorating; and when I use the term mental defect, I use it in connection with a condition not capable of either improving or deteriorating. I have used the term product of such mental disease or defect and causal connection between the condition of the criminal acts. The relationship must be such as to justify a reasonable inference that the acts would not have been committed if the accused had not been suffering from the disease or defect. These are the key factors; namely, a mental disease or defect and the relationship between that disease or defect and the criminal acts.

If the disease produces a mental derangement of such a character which necessarily influenced the defendant's action, there is no problem and the relationship between that disease or defect and the criminal acts. When the disease is of a lesser scope, the problem is not so simple.

The fact that the defendant had a mental disease or defect at the time of the crime is not sufficient, then to relieve him of responsibility of the crime. There must be a relationship between the disease or defect and the criminal act, and the relationship must be such as to justify a reasonable inference that the act would not have been committed if the person had not been suffering from such disease or defect.

By product of the disease, I do not mean that it must be a direct emission or a proximate creation or immediate issue of the disease. I do not mean to restrict the defense of insanity to such cases. I mean to say that the facts as found must be such that the jury is enabled to draw a reasonable inference that the accused would not have committed the acts, if he did commit them, if he had not been diseased as he was. These and that relationship, whatever it might be in degree, must be critical in respect of the acts.

By critical I mean decisive, determinative, causative. I mean to convey the idea inherent in the phrases, because of or except for, without which, but for, effect of, result of, causative factor, and that the disease made the effective or decisive difference between doing and not doing the act. This phrase, product of, is not intended to be precise, but means that the facts concerning the disease or the facts concerning the acts are such as to justify reasonably the conclusion that but for the disease the acts would not have been committed.

Now, what I have said is in some respects the manner of stating the defense, but as I have told you and shall hereafter state to you the burden of proof in respect to this defense is on the government, and the issue to be put to you is whether the government has met this defense beyond a reasonable doubt; that is, the jury must find beyond a reasonable doubt in order to return a verdict of guilty notwithstanding the defense of insanity that the accused is free of mental disease or defect, or, if finding that he has a mental disease or defect, that no relationship existed between the disease or defect and the alleged criminal acts which would justify the conclusion that but for the mental disease or defect the acts would not have been committed.

Therefore, if you believe beyond a reasonable doubt either that he was not suffering from a mental disease or defect, or if he was that the criminal acts were not the product of such abnormality, you may convict if you have found him to be otherwise guilty under the facts and the intructions I previously gave you before I started the instruction with respect to the defense of insanity.

If you do not believe beyond a reasonable doubt that the defendant was not suffering from a mental disease or defect or if he was that the criminal acts were not the product of such abnormality, then you must find him not guilty by reason of insanity." U.S. v. Oscar M. Ray, Jr., Crim. No. 250-61, given on May 24, 1962, Official Transcript of Proceedings, at 3-20.

In Case No. 3 the jury was charged *inter alia* as follows:

There is evidence in this case to the effect that the defendant did not have the mental capacity to commit the crimes with which she is charged because she was not mentally responsible for the acts committed.

Now, the law presumes that every person is sane, until the contrary appears. This presumption is based on human experience.

However, this does not mean that the burden of proof is on the defendant to prove insanity.

As soon as some evidence of mental disorder is offered in evidence, the presumption of sanity vanishes from the case, and the burden is then on the prosecution, or on the government, to establish the sanity of the accused beyond a reasonable doubt. In other words, on the issue of sanity, just as on every other issue in the case, the burden of proof is on the prosecution, and sanity, like any other fact, must be proved as part of the prosecution's case beyond a reasonable doubt.

The law in this jurisdiction states that those who of their own free will and with evil intent commit acts which violate the law shall be criminally responsible for those acts, but that where such acts stem from and are the product of a mental disease or defect, there is no legal responsibility.

The word "disease" is used in the sense of a condition which is considered capable of either improving or deteriorating, in other words, of growing worse. "Defect" is used in the sense of a condition which is not capable of either improving or deteriorating, and which may be either congenital, that is, existing at birth, or the result of injury, or the residual effect of a physical disease.

The law does not say that every person who suffers from a disease or a defective mental condition is excused from the legal consequences of an unlawful act he may commit. Only if the act was the product of a mental disease or defect can the accused be found not guilty on the ground of insanity.

Now, I have used the term product of such mental disease, or defect, and causal connection between the condition and the criminal act. This means that there must be a relationship between the condition and the criminal act. The relationship must be such as to justify a reasonable inference that the act would not have been committed if the accused had not been suffering from the disease or defect. These are the key factors, namely, a *mental disease or defect,* and the *relationship between that disease or defect and the criminal act.*

If the disease produces a mental derangement of such a character as necessarily to influence the defendant's actions, there is no problem as to the causal connection between the disease and the criminal act. When the disease is of a lesser scope, the problem is not so simple. The fact that a defendant had a mental disorder or defect at the time of the crime is not sufficient, then, to relieve him or her of responsibility for crime. There must be some relationship between the disease or defect and the criminal act, and the relationship must be such as to justify a reasonable inference that the act could not have been committed if the person had not been suffering from such disease.

By product of a disease, I do not mean that it must be a direct condition, or proximate creation or immediate issue of the disease. I do not mean to restrict the defense of insanity to such cases. I mean to say that the acts, if found, are such that the jury is unable to draw a reasonable inference that the accused would not have committed the acts, if she did commit them, if she had not been diseased as she was. There must be a relationship between the disease or defect and the act, and that relationship, whatever it might be in degree, must be critical in its effect with respect to the act.

Now, by critical I mean decisive, determinative, causative. I mean to convey the idea inherent in the phrase "because of," "except for," "but for which," "effect of," "causative factor," and the disease may be the effective or decisive difference between doing and not doing the act.

Now, the phrase 'product of' is not intended to be precise, but means that the facts concerning the disease, or the facts concerning the acts, are such as to justify reasonably the conclusion that but for the disease the act would not have been committed.

Mental abnormalities vary greatly in their nature and intensity and in their effect on the character and conduct of those who suffer from them. When a person suffering from a mental abnormality commits a crime, there is always a likelihood that the abnormality played some part in causing the crime; and, generally speaking, the more serious the abnormality, the more likely it is that the crime was caused by the mental disorder.

It is the jury's function to determine from all the evidence, including the expert testimony of the doctors, not only whether the defendant suffered from an abnormal mental condition at the time the crime was committed, but also whether the nature and extent of this condition was such as to have caused the defendant to do the unlawful act.

The problem for you is whether the accused was suffering from a mental disease or defect, that is, from a medically recognized illness of the mind; whether there was a relationship between special disease or defect and the specified alleged criminal act; and whether that relationship was such as to justify a reasonable inference that the accused would not have committed the act if she had the disease.

Now, what I have said is in no respect a matter of stating the defense, because I have told you and shall hereafter state to you that the burden of proof with respect to this defense is on the government, and the issue to be put to you is whether the government has met this defense beyond a reasonable doubt, that is, the jury must find beyond a reasonable doubt in order to convict, to return a verdict of guilty, notwithstanding the defense of insanity, that the accused is free from mental disease or defect, or a finding she may have a mental disease or defect if no relationship exists between the disease and the alleged criminal act which would justify the conclusion that but for the mental disease or defect the act would not have been committed.

Therefore, if you believe beyond a reasonable doubt either

that the defendant was not suffering from a disease or a mental defect, or a disease or a defective mental condition, or if she was, that the acts were not the product of such abnormality, you may convict if you find her to be otherwise guilty. U.S. v. Consuello Walker, Crim. No. 939-60, given May 26, 1961, Official Transcript of Proceedings, at 5-10. (Emphasis supplied).

APPENDIX III

At the time that the case described in Chapter 7 was tried —the then existing Harrison Narcotics Act prohibited, *inter alia,* the purchasing, selling, dispensing or distributing any narcotic drug—opium, Isonipecaine, coca leaves and other opiates and their derivatives except in "the original stamped package" evidencing payment of the excise tax. 26 U.S.C. 4704a (1954). It further prohibited selling, bartering, exchanging or giving away such drugs except pursuant to a written order prepared on forms supplied by the Treasury Department. Importers, manufacturers, wholesalers, pharmacists, physicians, etc., were required to register with the Treasury Department and to keep records available at all times for inspection by law enforcement officers.

Violations were penalized as follows:

A minimum sentence of two years for a first offense of possession of narcotics or marihuana, a minimum of five years for a second offense, and a minimum of ten years for any subsequent offense... A minimum of five years for a first offense of smuggling, selling, or otherwise transferring narcotics or marihuana, and a minimum of ten years for a second or subsequent offense. 26 U.S.C. 7237 (a) (1956).

Probation and parole were not available except in cases of a first offense for possession of narcotic drugs or marihuana. 26 U.S.C. 7237 (1956).

The recently amended Federal narcotics laws have not greatly changed the existing picture. To this day, the narcotics offender —be he a victim of his own addiction or a profiteer in the narcotics traffic—is subjected to extraordinary punishment.

The addict who has degenerated to a "down-and-outer" exclusively dependent on drug pushing to maintain his own supply —if he is to stave off dreaded withdrawal symptoms—is subjected to a welter of penalties which would seem to render any spy or murderer privileged by comparison. Thus the statute in dealing with the multiple offender—and a drug addict of some duration will invariably fall into this category—states that such an offender insofar as he is engaged "in a continuing criminal enterprise shall be sentenced to a term of imprisonment which may not be less than 10 years and which may be up to life imprisonment, to a fine of not more than $100,000, and to... forfeiture ... except that if any person engages in such activity after one or more prior convictions of him under this section have become final, he shall be sentenced to a term of imprisonment which may not be less than 20 years and which may be up to life imprisonment . . ." 21 U.S.C. §848 (1970).

Nor has anything been changed with regard to the prohibition of suspension of sentence and probation:

"In the case of any sentence imposed under this section, imposition or execution of such sentence shall not be suspended, probation shall not be granted." *Ibid.*

A half-hearted congressional attempt to provide for the noncriminal disposition of a case where the addict was engaged in selling to support his habit has not resulted in significant improvement of the lot of those handicapped by narcotics addiction. The available treatment facilities offered under Federal as well as State auspices are under-funded and lack the necessary psychological and material wherewithal to transform what would appear to be a coercive enterprise to a meaningful therapeutic program.

In *Watson* v. *United States,* 439 F.2d 442 (D.C. Cir. 1970) the Court of Appeals held that the two-year-felony disqualifying exclusion of Narcotic Addict Rehabilitation Act, creating a distinction between addicts who had trafficked in narcotics for the purpose of supporting their habit and non-trafficking addicts, guilty for the third time of possession of narcotics for their own use and hence declared ineligible for rehabilitative phase of the program was unconstitutional. But this in no way mitigated the enormity of the punishment otherwise visited on the offender and the Court did not seem swayed by the "cruel and unusual punishment" clause of the Constitution.